D. Gaenshirt, F. Harms, S. Rohmann, P. Schulz-Knappe

Peptidomics in Drug Development

Peptidomics
in Drug Development

Edited by

Dorothee Gaenshirt
Fred Harms
Sven Rohmann
Peter Schulz-Knappe

With contributions from

Annette Appel, Petra Budde, Gabriele Heine, Rüdiger Hess, Marco Jost, Michael Jürgens, Markus Kellmann, Jens Lamerz, Nicolas Le Yondre, Christoph Menzel, Susanne Neitz, Horst Rose, Michael Schrader, Martin U. Schuhmann, Imke Schulte, Hartmut Selle, Ranald Sutherland, Harald Tammen, Hans-Dieter Zucht

ECV Editio Cantor Verlag Aulendorf (Germany)

Bibliographic data available from the National Library of Germany ("Deutsche Bibliothek")

This publication is catalogued and indexed in "Deutsche Nationalbibliographie" of the National Library of Germany; detailed bibliographic data is available on the Internet at http://dnb.ddb.de

Peptidomics in Drug Development

ISBN 3-87193-323-6

Typeset by Texdo, Stuttgart (Germany); printed and bound by VeBu Druck + Medien GmbH, Bad Schussenried (Germany)

ECV · Editio Cantor Verlag on the Internet: www.ecv.de

Table of Contents

Introductory Note

Hanno Langen, MD

There is an increased need in the diagnostic and pharmaceutical industry for biomarkers. Proteomics technologies are offering the potential to discover new candidate biomarkers which then can be validated during the clinical phases of a drug development. Biomarkers play an important role in the pharmaceutical industry and become more and more important in drug discovery and development. The potential benefit of biomarkers is to allow earlier, more robust drug safety and efficacy measurement. Generally a better understanding of the mechanism of disease progression, response prediction and therapeutic intervention is needed and the concept of applying biomarkers early on in drug development becomes more and more evident. The standard technologies of proteomics are focused on proteins and not so much on naturally occurring peptides in the low molecular weight range below 10 kDa. This book is offering insights into technologies directed to discover these peptides and shows very interesting examples how the so called peptidomics technologies are used in the drug discovery process. These peptides can be naturally occurring peptide hormones like insulin or are breakdown products from larger proteins like albumin. The greatest challenge in peptidomics and proteomics is to overcome the huge dynamic expression difference of proteins and peptides, which can account for more than 10 orders of magnitude. Efficient removal of the proteins before analyzing the peptides can already overcome partially this challenge. In this book not only the technical challenges and solutions for them are described but also application in various disease areas. The application span areas like the diseases of the central nervous system, oncology and metabolic diseases. This book describes additional tools to generate candidate biomarker lists for many pharmaceutical applications which then can be validated by traditional immunological tests like ELISAs or others.

Peptidomics appears to have a bright future in drug development and the readers gain insights into the challenges and possible solutions, application of the new field of peptidomics, which was pioneered by the company BioVisioN.

Hoffmann-La Roche, Basel (Switzerland)
June 2005

Preface

Peter Schulz-Knappe, MD, PhD

The expectation of the public towards improved health care by advancement of science is high. To fulfil these expectations pharmaceutical as well as biotech industry spend enormous resources on the discovery and development of novel, better drugs. Over the last 5 years, a slight shift has occurred from „blockbuster" type drugs towards more targeted approaches. It would be feasible to already announce the beginning of the era of "personalised medicine", where patients are treated with a drug only if conclusive evidence exists that the patient would response in a favourable way. Nevertheless, today budgetary as well as knowledge restrictions (both imprinting heavily on each other) still make such cases the exemption, not the rule.

A core factor to further promote quality of drug treatment lies in the precise description of a drug's action, its side effects and adverse events, and its complex interaction with the individual patient. This factor goes "hand in hand" with a better understanding of the complexity of diseases, such as the diversity of diseases, and the time course of diseases, such as early detection that would demand different treatment options. With the appropriate data, a selection of drugs and treatment schemes for patients seems possible that would increase responder rates dramatically, meanwhile sparing those "non-responder" patients from possible side effects. As another crucial factor, time would be saved and appropriate alternatives to treat non responders could be selected much earlier than today. It is clear that these factors together would also have great socio-economical impact.

Over time, the number of drugs being prescribed only for selected patient populations will need to increase in order to meet such expectations. Given the continuously rising costs of drug development in an environment where health care spending seems to have reached a plateau, there is a deadlock scenario where it is no longer possible, from a financial perspective, to increase the number of new drugs simply by the fact that reimbursement would not lead to an adequate return on investment. Development costs have to come down. Development times have to be shortened. Drug candidates that enter into the expensive phases of clinical development have to be selected by appropriate measures to an extent that drastically reduces attrition rate.

We are positive that these aspects in drug development can be addressed and solved. An unsurpassed amount of information can be gained today by the use of modern science. Especially the many varieties of "omics" type technologies will help to elucidate molecular biology, epidemiology, individual disease and drug response, and lead to higher quality of drugs and/or better selection of that subpopulation of patients that will really benefit from treatment. Strikingly, it seems feasible that this can be achieved in shorter developmental times even if much more data are accumulated. One simple scenario may illustrate the potential: If, by the use of novel, scientific know-how, the pre-selection of patients to be enrolled into a phase III-clinical trial would lead to an increase in responder rate from 25 to 50 %, the number of patients needed to reach regulatory maturity is drastically reduced. This would lead to great savings in cost and developmental time.

A novel way to obtain such valuable data is presented in this book. Peptidomics is defined as the systematic, comprehensive analysis of peptides of a biological sample at a defined timepoint and location. Peptides (small proteins) are biomolecules that occur in all body fluids such as blood and urine, and in cells and tissues. Since peptides reflect the activity of genes, proteins, enzymes and overall metabolism in health and disease, they are useful to diagnose diseases, to improve the understanding of disease development and treatment. Peptides are ideal biomarkers.

We describe in this book several applications of peptidomics technologies for biomedical research that are capable of improving drug development. A variety of biomarker studies on cells, tissues and human blood samples are presented that describe the technology in detail. This part of the book is rather directed towards researchers. We have also tried to address those readers that are more interested in the economical impact of peptidomics. In that part, the first global primary data evaluation is presented that was performed among the top pharmaceutical companies. The investigation reflects the current importance and future perspectives of peptidomics in drug development.

The authors believe that the great progress in life sciences over the last decade has just begun, opening the field for further research and advancement in medical science. The novel research field "peptidomics" will contribute to continuous improvement of health in the future.

BioVisioN, Hannover (Germany)
June 2005

1 The World of Peptidomics

1.1 Introduction

Peter Schulz-Knappe
and Sven Rohmann

Drug discovery as well as early- and late stage development of drugs and biomarkers are in a continuous adaptation and maturation process. The cycle of significant changes based on new findings is coupled with shifts in research priorities and continues to make this part of pharmaceutical research a most challenging endeavour.

Over the last years, the emphasis on genomics has shifted via transcriptomics to proteomics, the science of understanding how proteins in their entirety actually translate gene information into function at the cellular level, and metabonomics, the science of small molecular, non-polymer entities that are further apart from genomic work than any other of the "omics" type of approaches.

Proteomics, which already has gained the character of a buzzword within the last 6-8 years, describes the analysis of the protein complement of a biological sample with respect to temporal and spatial resolution. This technology field is mainly based on separation of complex protein mixtures by two-dimensional gel electrophoresis with gel digests and mass spectrometric analysis of the extracted protein fragments or, recently evolving with increasing popularity, on multi-step chromatographical approaches, usually combined with protease digestion of proteins. This is a technical manoeuvre performed at different stages of the analysis process to serve the sole purpose of facilitating handling, separation, and identification of the complex protein set-up of the samples.

Proteomics has recently been flanked by peptidomics, a new direction in proteomic research aiming at the comprehensive visualisation and analysis of small polypeptides in the molecular mass range of 1 to 20 kDa, thus covering the gap between proteomics and metabonomics, with some overlap to both areas. The refinement of peptidomics is based on an essential paradigm related to modularity and diversity in gene product function. Peptides are a paramount example of how nature diversifies from one single gene to release multiple, regulated functionalities at the desired sites and at the desired time.

To achieve this, peptides are sequentially generated by a complex network of more than 500 proteases, acting at intracellular sites, upon secretion, in extracellular environments, and, finally, serving (regulated) degradation. This cycle of maturation, activation and degradation is best considered as an irreversible in vivo reaction.

Due to the evolving technologies in peptidomics, we can expect fast and relevant progress in understanding protein and peptide networks from a systems biology approach leading to the discovery of multiple new diagnostic and therapeutic targets. However, the way from a complex biological sample such as a body fluid, a cell extract, or tissue to identification of potential targets will heavily depend on technological developments and on the ability to adequately analyse well powered studies to differentiate between true disease related signals and false positive ones and to identify false negative signals. Subsequently, validation of findings will be the next hurdle moving target discovery further to target validation, which will be the next value-driver for this research field.

This book aims at an overview of peptidomics technologies by collecting a variety of applications from pioneering work performed at BioVisioN AG (Hannover, Germany) in the years 1997 to 2004. Also a primary data evaluation among global pharmaceutical R&D experts is included that was performed by the Health Care Competence Centre HC3 (Basel, Switzerland) addressing the impact of peptidomics on pharmaceutical drug development.

1.2 The Post-Genomics Era

Peter Schulz-Knappe and Michael Schrader

During the completion of the human proteome, a wide variety of additional "omics" technologies arose, most of them dealing with comprehensive analysis of distinct groups of biomolecules. Well established at this stage is transcriptomics as a high-throughput technology to profile gene expression in a certain cell or tissue type. It is used to classify compounds and to profile a drug's action on a global scale, displaying the changes in a subset of genes. It has to be noted that protein expression may not correlate well with mRNA levels, since not only the rate of biosynthesis but also the speed of the degradation processes of mRNAs and proteins determine the abundance of a certain protein.

The rather long way from genotype to phenotype is further analysed using proteomics, peptidomics and metabolomics. These technologies are further complemented by pharmacogenomics and nutrigenomics, which address the influence of drugs and nutrition. In general, we can subsume all these technologies as members of the post-genomics era (Fig. 1). In addition, there exists a wide variety of flavours also using "omics" approaches, such as glycomics, lipomics, cellomics, degradomics and so on, that contribute to the field. There seem to be multiple applications for these technologies, either alone or in combination, and we believe that a "Systems Biology" approach will strongly benefit from integrating their analytical power.

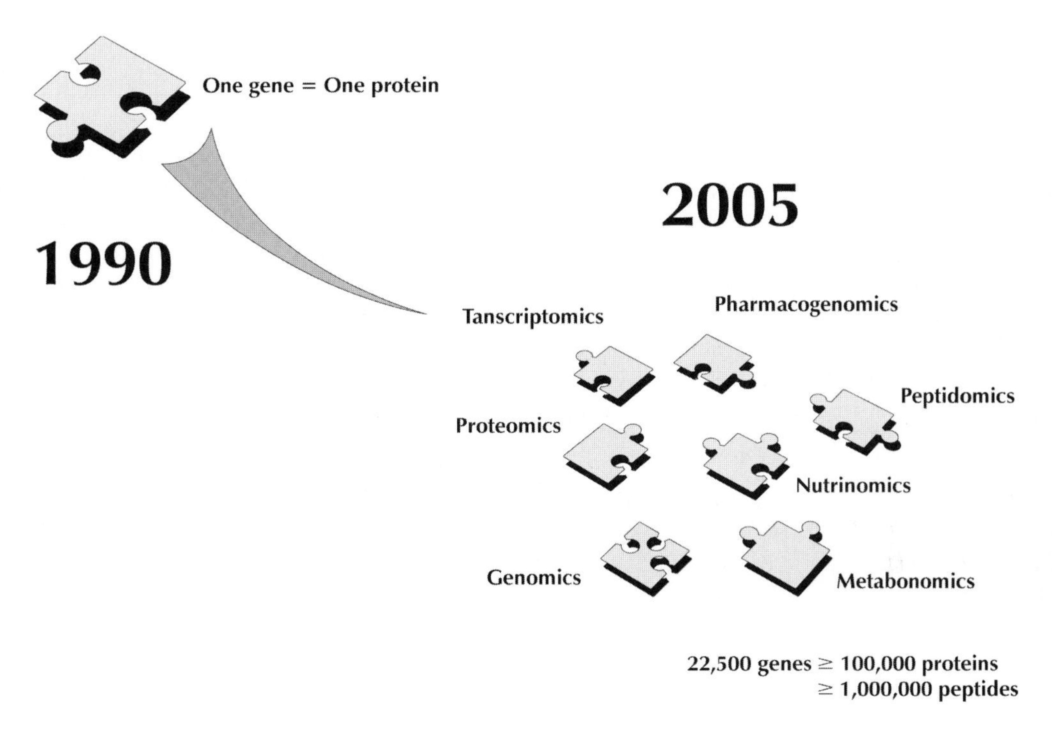

Fig. 1: The post-genomics era.
The original concept of the 90th „one gene – one protein – one function" has changed dramatically during and after the completion of the human genome. Several „omics"type technologies now face the challenge to integrate enormous amounts of divergent data into biological knowledge.

Peptidomics is defined as the systematic, comprehensive analysis of peptides of a biological sample at a defined timepoint and location.

In the first part of the book, we want to summarise the application of peptidomics technologies for biomedical research and drug development. We have selected a variety of "proof of principle" studies that shall describe technical issues relevant for successful studies and we detailed the analysis of blood samples. This is, to our knowledge, one of the most difficult tasks in peptidomics analysis, since the plasma proteome is the most diverse and the "deepest" proteome in terms of the differences in analyte concentration. In Fig. 2; see page 18, a collection of events is given that participate in the regulation of peptide and protein composition in the circulation. Note that there are time- and location-dependent effects that affect either biosynthesis or maturation of protein precursors before they reach a mature, bioactive form. As well, the life cycle of peptides and proteins is again regulated by numerous events, which themselves seem to be strictly regulated by localised and well-timed events such as proteolysis, diffusion, excretion, binding and reuptake, and lysosomal degradation, just to name a few of them.

Systemic Circulation

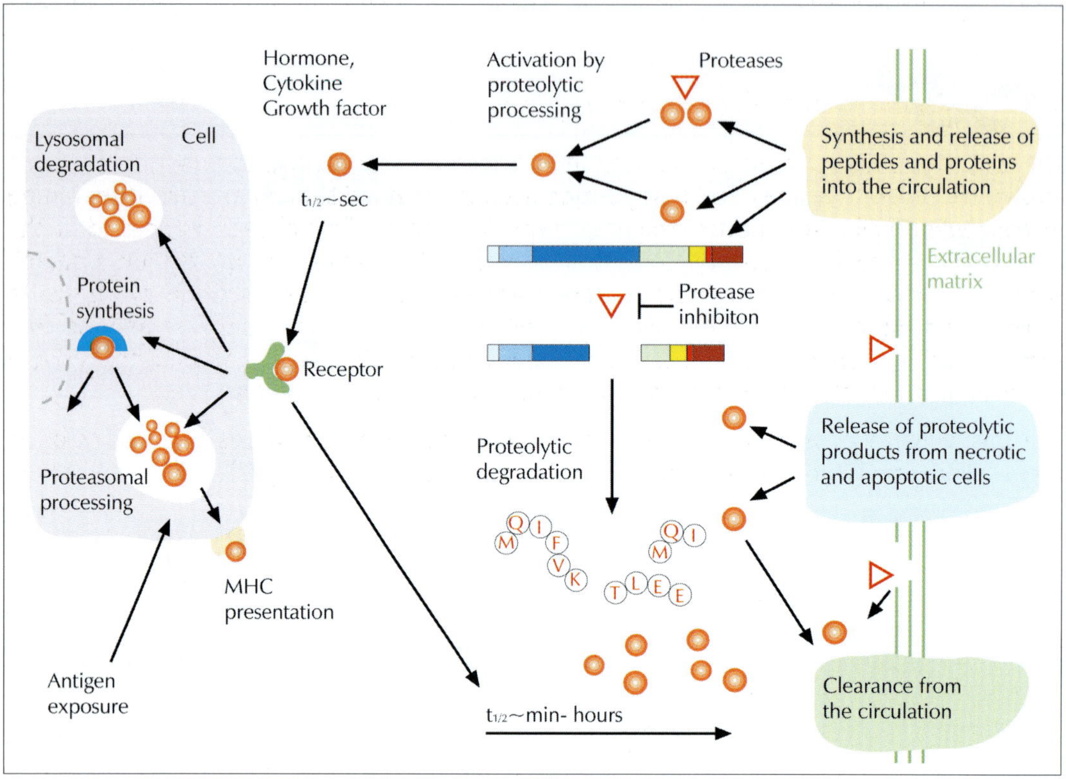

Fig. 2: Peptide generation, bioactivity and degradation.
A brief illustration on the multiplicity of events feeding the peptidome. Input as well as output is regulated by biochemical and physicochemical processes that explain in part the highly dynamic composition of peptides in biological samples.

In the following chapter we want to present the first global primary data evaluation that was performed among pharmaceutical R&D experts in European, US-American, and Japanese pharmaceutical companies actively involved in peptidomics. This investigation reflects the current importance and future perspectives of peptidomics in drug development focusing the degree to which it will influence certain R&D areas and major indications. Ultimately, the study reveals the commitment of the pharmaceutical industry to this technology. In addition, superiorities and inherent disadvantages of peptidomics are discussed and future methodological steps to take are indicated by pharmaceutical experts.

The authors of this book believe that the great progress in life sciences over the last decade has just begun to open the field for further research and advancement in medical science. We anticipate that relevant discoveries will be made in the future and that they will lead to continuous improvement of health. We are convinced that the novel research field "peptidomics" will contribute to this development, and we present an outlook of peptidomics in the last chapter of this book.

1.3 Peptides of Pharmaceutical Relevance

Peter Schulz-Knappe

1.3.1 Peptides in biology and medicine

The role of peptides in biology and their importance for therapeutic applications has been known for several decades. The first peptide used to treat a disabling and life-threatening disease was insulin for the treatment of type 1 diabetes. This already happened in the beginning of the last century. Closely accompanied by advances in peptide research such as Edman degradation for sequence analysis, solid phase peptide synthesis to provide synthetic material and basic as well as advanced methods for peptide and protein purification such as HPLC, many more peptides with biological importance were discovered of which quite some contribute to today's medical practise.

The involvement of peptides in distinct disease areas, either as drugs themselves or as target points at which drug therapy is directed, is impressive (Fig. 3). Indications range

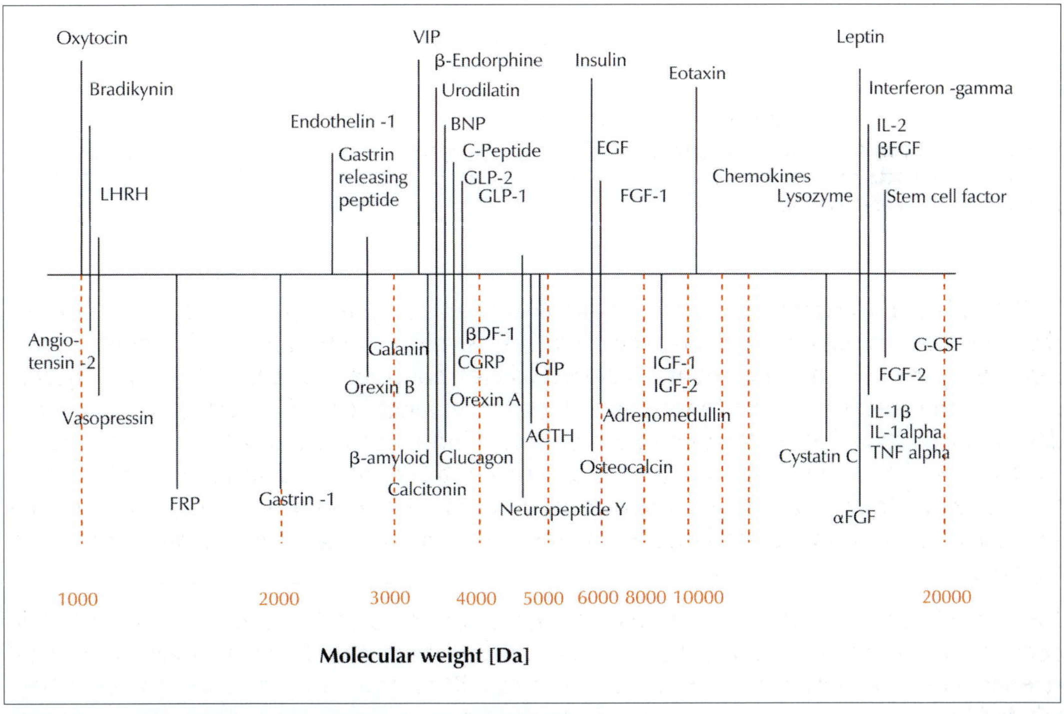

Fig. 3: Selected biologically active peptides and small proteins.
Endogenous peptides that are involved in numerous physiological functions are sorted on a "peptidomics mass scale" from 1,000 to 20,000Da according to the molecular weight of the biologically active peptide.

from oncology via neurodegeneration, osteoporosis, blood pressure regulation, blood glucose and fat metabolism to fertility and immunology. Table 1 summarises a few examples of peptide blockbuster drugs with respect to their economic potential. So far we were not able to pinpoint a disease area *without* involvement of peptides in a central manner. Thus, peptides play a pivotal role as indicators of disease as biomarkers or diagnostics. To illustrate this, Table 2 lists some peptide based biomarkers and diagnostics. The large collection of areas in biology and medicine with proven direct and powerful peptide involvement makes it necessary to address this class of biomolecules with the appropriate technologies for discovery and development both from a scientific as well as from a commercial perspective.

Trade name	Compound	Company	Indication
Humulin	Insulin	Eli Lilly	Diabetes
Betaseron	Interferon-β	Schering	Multiple sclerosis
Forteo	Parathyroid hormone	Eli Lilly	Osteoporosis
Gonal-F	Follicle-stimulating hormone	Serono	Fertility
Sandimmune	Cyclosporine	Novartis	Transplant rejection
Zoladex	Synthetic peptide of LHRH	AstraZeneca	Prostate cancer
Natrecor	hBNP	Scios	Heart failure
Copaxone	Four amino acids from myelin	Teva/Aventis	Multiple sclerosis
Zestril	Synthetic peptide derivative of ACE inhibitor	AstraZeneca	Hypertension

Table 1: Peptide therapeutics.

Peptide	Molecular mass [kDa]	Disease
Insulin	5.7	Diabetes
C-peptide	3.1	Diabetes
Proinsulin	9.5	Diabetes
Brain natriuretic peptide (BNP)	3.5	Congestive heart failure
and N-terminal-pro BNP (NT-proBNP)	8.5	
Amyloid Aβ 1-40	4.1	Alzheimer's disease
Amyloid Aβ 1-42	4.3	Alzheimer's disease
Trypsinogen-activating peptide (TAP)	0.9	Pancreatitis
Procalcitonin (PCT)	14	Bacterial infection/sepsis
β-2 Microglobulin	12	Renal failure
Osteocalcin	5.8	Osteoporosis
Cystatin C	13	Renal failure

Table 2: Peptide based diagnostics and biomarkers.

1.4 How are Peptides Produced and Processed?

Hans-Dieter Zucht

1.4.1 Introduction

Peptides like proteins contain amino acid residues connected by peptides bonds that are considered as fairly stable under physiological conditions. Their sizes range from a few up to some 150 amino acid residues. Since there exists no clear cut definition for the term "peptide" to distinguish it from the term protein, we refer to peptides in a range from dipeptides to peptides with a molecular mass < 20kDa, therefore small proteins may be included in our definition. The linear coding template for any peptide primary structure sequence is found in the genome. The origin of the word peptide is *peptein,* the Greek word for "to digest", or *pepsis* for digestion, introduced by the German chemist Emil Fischer (who has been awarded the Nobel Prize in chemistry in 1902), reminding us that peptides are usually generated by digestion (Fig. 4). This chapter will focus on the mechanisms that are responsible for the formation of peptides within higher organisms, and describe which factors – especially proteases – are determining peptide structure and peptide concentration.

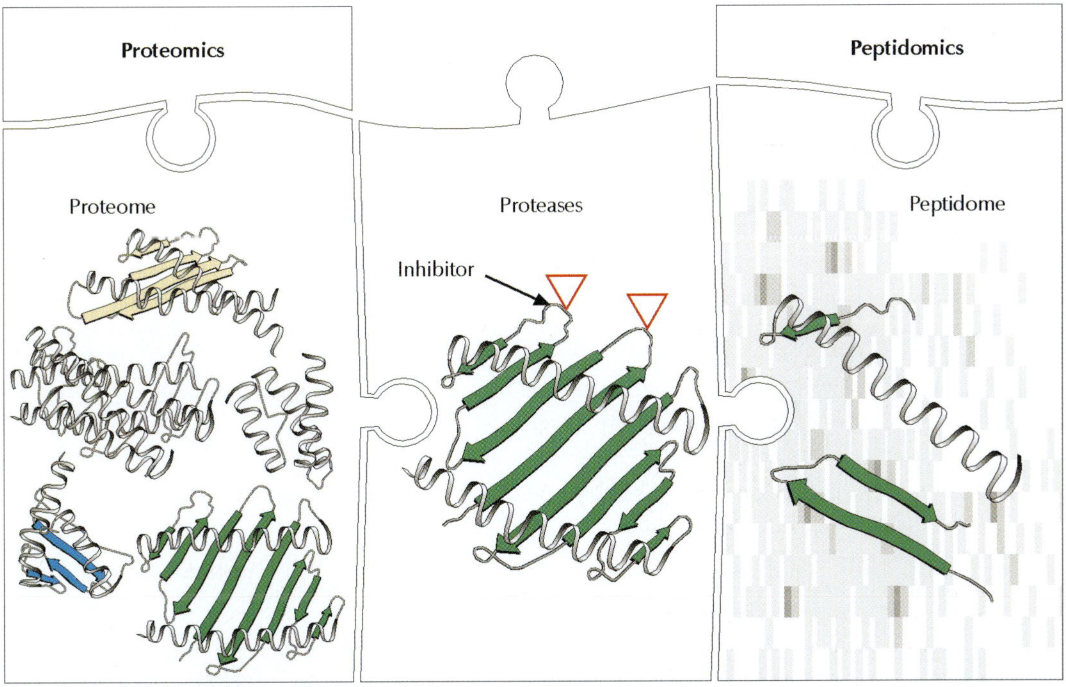

Fig. 4: Proteomics and peptidomics belong to post-genome technologies.

The proteome and the peptidome are complex settings that change with respect to location and time. Proteases and their inhibitors play a key role in the conversion of proteins to peptides, thus balancing proteome and peptidome.

1.4.2 Molecular biology

Peptides in a biological compartment can be described by their exact molecular nature, and one basis of this is the amino acid sequence. This primary structure allows the alignment of a peptide sequence with mRNA and finally with the corresponding genomic DNA sequences. The profiling of peptide patterns in vivo usually reveals a large variety of peptides in every biological compartment. Not uncommon, a multiplicity of peptides can be clustered together originating from the same protein precursor.

There is a well accepted information hierarchy among biopolymers involved in each living organism. The genomic DNA is considered as the information template which is transcribed into mRNA and further translated into the precursors of proteins and peptides (Fig. 5).

In the early days of molecular biology, the concept was that one gene is coding for one protein which is responsible for one function. The contemporary biochemistry dramatically changed this picture. During protein biosynthesis, a large amount of variability is possible.

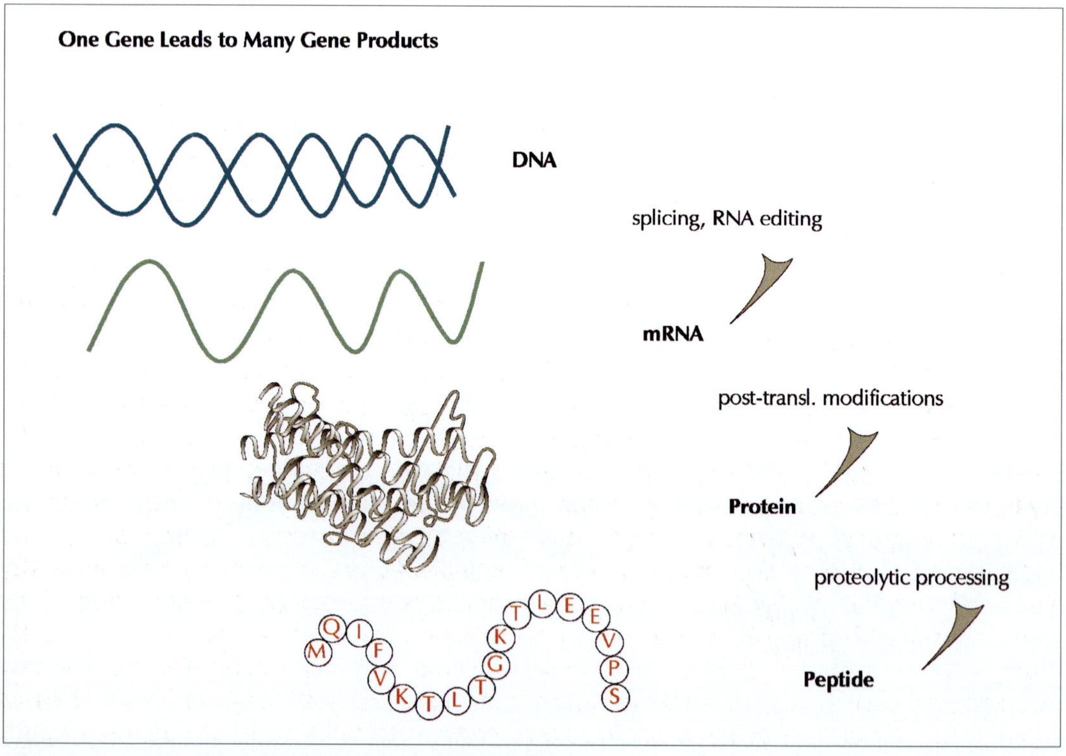

Fig. 5: Information hierarchy from genotype to phenotype.
Tightly regulated multi-step events convert genomic information via RNA and proteins into peptides.

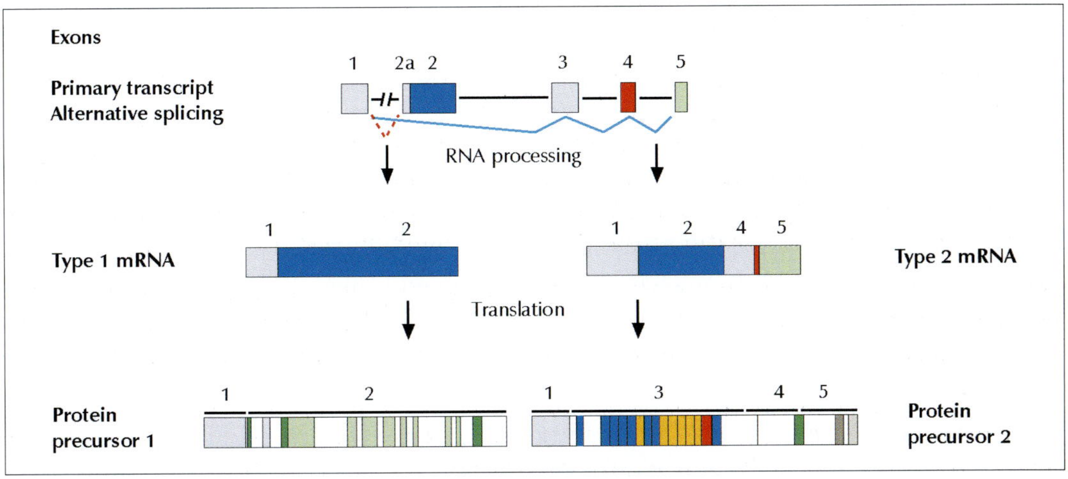

Fig. 6: The FMRF system.

The FMRF amide gene in the species Lymnea is a popular example for a gene translated by a complex information flow from the gene to the final peptide precursor proteins. One gene leads to different mRNAs due to alternative splicing. Each of the resulting precursor proteins contains many different biologically active peptides depicted with different colours.

Alternative splicing, exon skipping, and post-translational modifications are a few relevant examples within the route of protein and peptide generation. The processing of peptides adds up for possible diversity. One single gene can give rise to a large variety of peptides, derived from proteolysis and post-translational modifications, which are structurally and functionally different.

An example of a peptide system which has been thoroughly investigated, describing such a complex cascade of peptide formation, is the FMRF amide system present in organisms such as the freshwater snail Lymnea (Fig. 6). The FMRF system is phylogenetically very old, showing the complex regulatory possibilities and access points (e.g. gene regulation, splicing mechanisms, protein processing, gene dosage) for peptide biosynthesis. Such type of peptide precursors can be considered as containers holding multiple – initially hidden – functionalities. Usually, it is observed that these cryptic peptides are liberated by highly specific proteases such as prohormone convertases (PC). On the other hand, we know proteolytical processes in organisms which are less specific. For example, during ingestion of milk protein, a large variety of biologically active peptides are transiently liberated from the milk protein casein, such as opioid peptides or peptide antibiotics. They certainly serve distinct, beneficial biological functions such as regulation of intestinal flora, sleepiness of the suckling after breast feeding and many more. One may follow the concept that it is of evolutionary benefit if degradation of larger proteins releases distinct functionalities. It is no surprise that certain domains of serum albumin might contain antimicrobial properties that might be produced in considerable amounts at the protease-rich site of bacterial infection.

1.4.3 Peptide metabolism and processing

Almost every peptide found in higher organisms has its origin in the processing of a larger (protein/peptide) precursor. This means that for the generation of any peptide, there are dedicated processes involved that tailor the precursor through a series of events. Proteolysis of peptide bonds is catalysed by specific enzymes called peptidases or proteases. Because of alterations in peptidase composition and concentration, the concentration of many peptides, together forming peptide patterns, change dynamically. The multiplex way of reactions is itself regulated by a multiplicity of peptidase inhibitors. The interaction of peptides with peptidases can virtually create an almost infinitive number of possible peptide structures, whereas only a limited number is usually observed in vivo.

Research on *peptidases* and their inhibitors covers the main principle factors responsible for peptide processing and thus for the exact primary structures that are observed in a peptidome.

Peptidases that cleave internal peptide bonds of a given polypeptide substrate are called *endopeptidases*. Their action usually releases two resulting fragment peptides. In contrast to this mode of action, *exopeptidases* process polypeptides by (consecutively) liberating amino acids from the N- or C-terminus, thus leading to truncated products. Any of these proteolytic events creates novel peptide termini, and it is important that all these peptides now have to be considered as individuals, and they may carry an own, unique type of information. Peptide cleavage usually results in decrease or increase of the actual biological activity of the peptide, in some cases it can lead to biological activity different from the previous activity.

The specific interaction of a peptide with a peptidase requires specific molecular interactions. Usually, the reactions are guided by the presence of certain defined amino acid residues. As a consequence, the reaction catalysed by a peptidase has a given sequence specificity. The hydrolytical reaction itself is energetically favourable, the equilibrium usually lies far on the side of the products. The susceptibility of substrates for proteases determines the reaction speed, which is related to the activity of the protease and the accessibility of the cleavage site of the polypeptide substrate. Important examples for peptide releasing mechanisms are the removal of the secretory signal peptides, the removal of pro-pieces during peptide maturation or peptide formation by nonspecific degradation of proteins.

A change of only a single amino acid residue might already have a significant influence on a peptide's physicochemical nature resulting in different functions. In some occasions, peptides of slightly different lengths share functional properties with different degrees of bioactivity. For example, insulin is synthesized in the pancreas as a prohormone where an internal peptide (C-peptide) is cleaved off and the residual dibasic residues are removed by carboxypeptidase activity (Fig. 8; see page 27). Eventually, insulin is degraded by insulin degrading enzymes. Usually, only mature insulin is considered as the relevant bioactive part, but it is described that the prohormone as well as C-peptide have certain bioactivities, an observation which may also be true for other molecular forms. There are other examples illustrating this principle: GLP-1 receptor agonists and antagonists differ only in their length. Molecular variants exist for numerous peptide hormones such as CCK, PACAP or somatostatin. Another well-known example for complex peptide processing is described for the cerebral peptide hormone precursor proopio-melanocortin. The precursor is cleaved by proteases releasing several different peptide hormones, such as ACTH, lipotropin, alpha-MSH, ß-MSH, and endorphin. All these released hormones play a certain role in analgesia and stress response, indicating that the synthesis of the POMC precursor is meaningful in certain common physiological situations. Individual peptides have specific half-lives that are already determined by their primary structure. The processing of the precursor protein into the many different peptides is performed by a set of peptidases that show tissue specific distribution in the various parts of the hypophyseal gland. Thus, true differential processing occurs, enabling the organism to adapt to exogenous or endogenous stimuli at several levels.

1.4.4 The role of peptidases in peptide processing

The human genome contains a considerably high number of genes for proteases and peptidases. The MEROPS database currently describes 504 entries of proteases which account for 2.5% of the approx. 22,500 human genes. In addition, a large number of protease inhibitors is encoded. They are usually high abundant proteins that are competing substrates. The database contains information about protease families on the basis of sequence specificity and structure. Proteases are classified according to the nature of the active site as aspartic proteases, cysteine proteases, threonine proteases, metalloproteinases, or serine proteases. Some of them are highly specific cleaving only one single substrate. For example, coagulation factor X only cleaves thrombin in the coagulation cascade at the site of Ile-Glu-Gly-Arg. Other proteases are restricted to process a limited number of substrates. The intracellular prohormone convertases cleave a variety of protein substrates shortly after their synthesis. The family of prohormone convertases (PCs) of the subtilisin-kexin like family (Fig. 7, see page 26) contains 8 known members of proteases. The PCs 1-7 cleave protein substrates during their synthesis in the golgi apparatus, whereas furin is located in the cell membrane. The proteases PC1, PC2, furin, PACE4, PC4, PC5, and PC7 process precursors at the C-terminal residue of singly and paired basic amino acid residues. In contrast, SKI-1 cleaves proproteins at hydrophobic residues. The proteases PC1 and PC2 are assumed to be responsible for the processing of most endocrine and neuroendocrine precursors. The other proteases process proteins formed in a constitutive secretory pathway.

The substrates of prohormone convertases contain basic amino acid residues at the cleavage site. This is a prerequisite for cleavage because the preferred locations of prohormone convertase cleavage sites are dibasic sites (Fig. 8, see page 27). There are further preferences for cleavage at certain sequence positions that contain specific motifs based on certain amino acid constellations. When analysing a precursor protein which contains several dibasic sites, not all sites are utilised for processing in all cell types that express the precursor protein. It is therefore necessary to investigate which peptides are preferentially liberated in vivo.

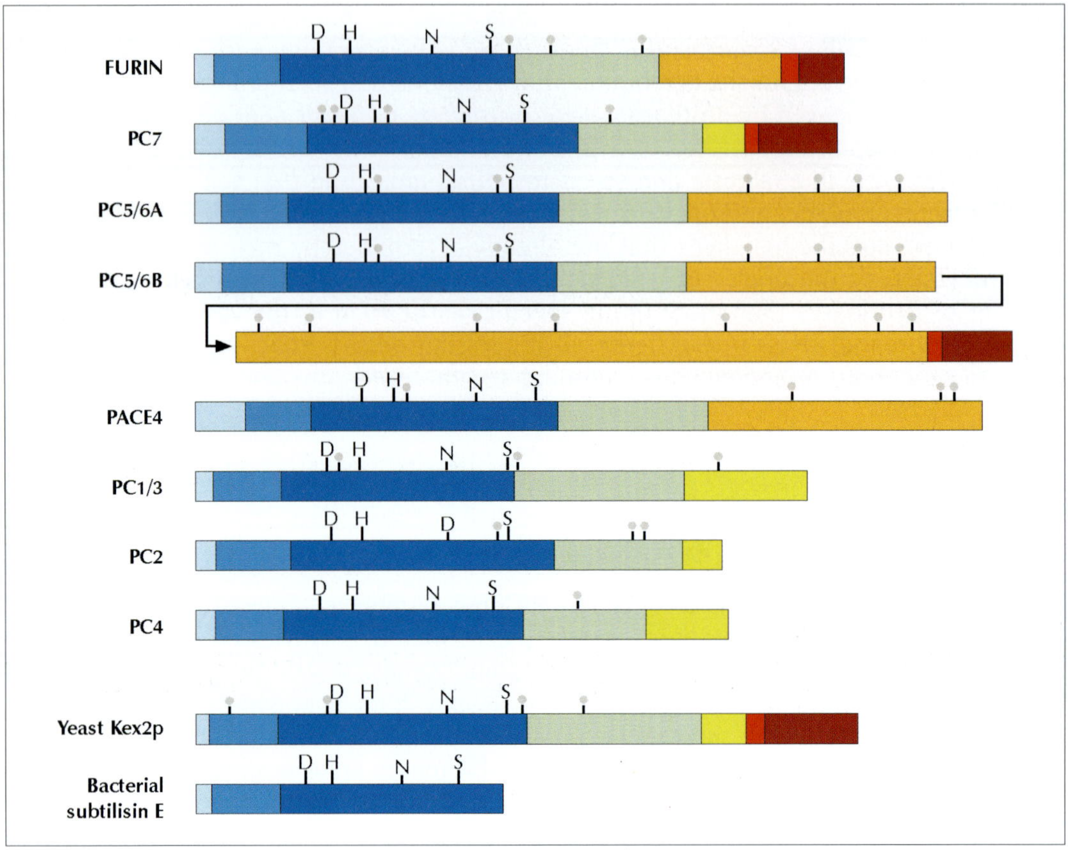

Fig. 7: The subtilisin/kexin like family of prohormone convertases.

The subtilisin/kexin like family of prohormone convertases share a common modular organization. The modules are depicted in light blue: signal peptide, mid blue: prodomain, dark blue: subtilisin like catalytic domain, green: P-domain, orange: Cys rich domain, yellow: Ser/Thr rich region, red: transmembrane domain, dark red: cytoplasmic domain.

In many cases, the prediction of the molecular form of native peptides is not easily achieved by computational approaches. For example, the N- and C-termini of many processed peptides are modified by post-translational processes such as N-terminal pyroglutamic acid formation and C-terminal amidation. Such type of modification usually leads to a stabilization of the peptide, removing the susceptibility toward the action of exopeptidases, indicating that the peptide contains a valuable functionality which is relevant for the organism. Many peptide hormones, in particular in the brain, show modifications of this type.

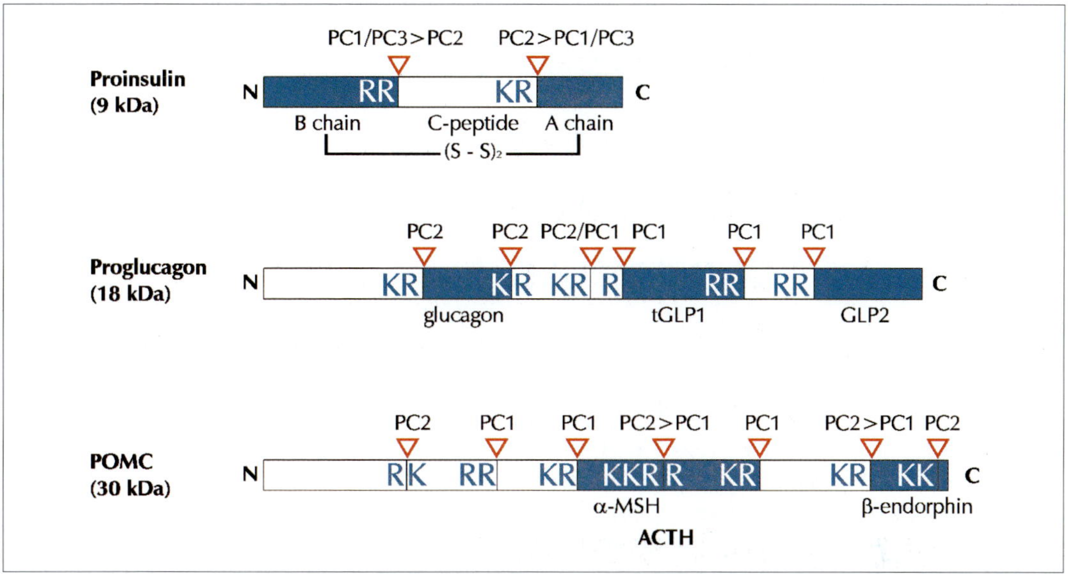

Fig. 8: Prohormone convertase processing sites.
Localization of prohormone convertase (PC) processing sites in the precursor proteins of proinsulin, proglucagon and POMC (red triangles). Each cleavage site contains two essential basic residues (K: Lysine, R: Arginine) and has a defined susceptibility being cleaved by the prohormone convertases PC1, PC2 and PC3.

Protease inhibitors are another essential part of these complex metabolic networks. Non specific protease inhibitors protect the organism against unwanted proteolytic events. Most compartments have "global protection systems", an integral part of which are protease inhibitors. Plasma for example is known to possess a high degree of trypsin inhibiting activity suitable for an attenuation of many proteolytic systems. Proteolytic events are usually transient events, and these are often related to pathophysiology. A lack of antitrypsin, for example, is a severe pathological condition, associated with dramatic pulmonary consequences.

A further general principle for the production of peptides shall be mentioned. The proteasome machinery of each cell is a special system capable of delivering enormous amounts and a high diversity of peptides. This fact is often neglected, when discussing peptide biochemistry. It is estimated that 25% or more of normal as well as defective protein biosynthesis are directly shuttled towards the proteasome, so one may conclude that proteasome derived peptides will give a fairly good representation of the input to the cellular proteome. The reaction which triggers the subjection of proteins to the proteasome is the ubiquitinylation. This is a reversible modification that targets a protein for a variety of fates including the degradation by the proteasome.

As a result, every cell contains a large number of intracellular peptides derived from the degradation of a certain proportion of the whole proteome, short peptides are created which are presented by the MHC complex at the cell surface and which have a primary structure following certain defined processing rules. This peptide epitope display is a process which links the interaction of the immune system with the proteome of cells triggering immune reactions.

1.4.5 Outlook

As a result, a biological function is distributed between a variety of molecules, connected with each other by metabolic reactions. The multiplicity of reactions connecting the individual concentration pools can be considered as a metabolomic network, where it is hard to point on singular particles with a given function. The final concentration results from the balance of these reactions. As a result, the concentration of any given peptide mirrors many physiological events: protein synthesis, secretion, proteolysis, degradation, diffusion, and also pathophysiological effects in the organism. As a result, the peptide concentration is a function of time and physiological conditions, which is the reason why peptides are useful as biomarkers in medical research.

To our surprise, current molecular biology revealed quite a limited number of genes in the human genome. By the end of 2004, the number of human genes has successively dropped from initial estimates of >100,000 to an estimated number of 22,500 genes. Moreover, scientists learned that some less complex, less diverse organisms had more, or proportionally more, genes than human beings. This lack of correlation between genome size and an organism's complexity raised the question how complexity and diversity arise in higher life forms. The concept of peptidomics investigating peptides, proteases, their inhibitors, and biological function is one way to remind us of how many different functional concepts can be hidden in one single gene. The system state of a peptidome (e.g. the structures and concentration of peptides found) is the consequence of the participating metabolic processes and has to be considered as plastic and highly susceptible towards post-translational modifications.

1.5 General Outline of Peptidomics Technologies

Peter Schulz-Knappe, Hartmut Selle, Hans-Dieter Zucht, and Michael Schrader

Initially, in the late 1980's the vision existed, that a collection of suitable technologies would be capable to explore the large *"terra incognita"* of peptides in living organisms. Fueled by the background of known bioactive peptides like insulin, there was quite some enthusiasm that the knowledge about this group of compounds is exceptionally useful in medical research. This view was fostered by the constantly growing knowledge on peptides, like their high diversity in living systems and their involvement in key regulatory processes. A need for improved peptide discovery, ideally combining peptide sequence identification with peptide profiling, emerged in order to find new peptides relevant as biomarkers and proto-peptide drugs. Such an approach would allow to systematically analyse peptide patterns in a given sample matrix, compare different patterns relating to specific metabolic or pathologic conditions and identify peptides of interest, i.e. compounds which show a potential as a biomarker. Standard proteomic approaches were not suitable for a systematic peptide analysis, since they do not cover peptides, the group of low molecular weight proteins (Fig. 9). The sizes of these biomolecules range between those of metabolites and proteins, and can indeed be addressed as *terra incognita* reflecting the largely unexplored nature of this field.

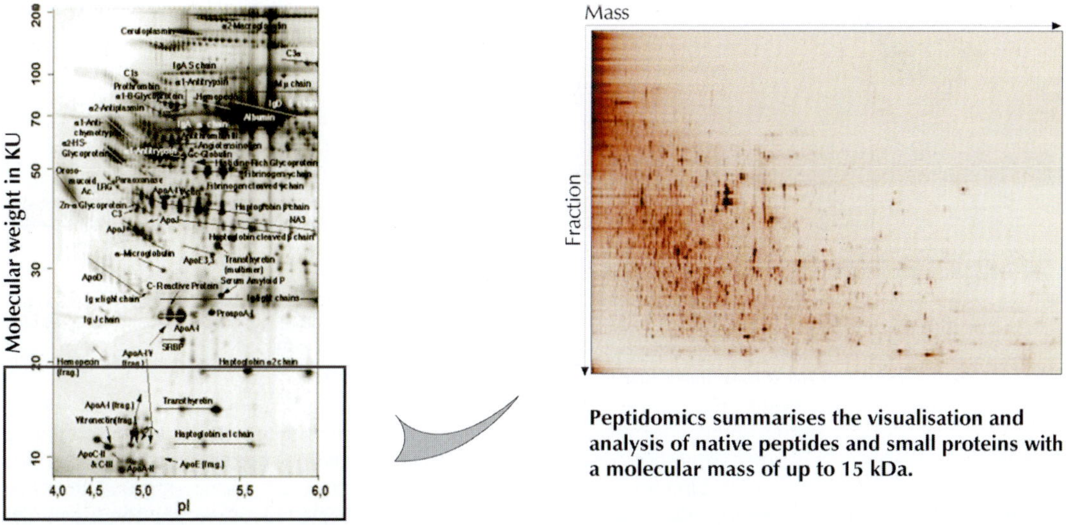

Fig. 9: The low molecular weight proteome can be discovered with peptidomics.

As a consequence, specific *peptidomics* technologies have been developed addressing sample preparation and reduction of sample complexity, sensitive analytical detection by mass spectrometry, sequence determination, and differential analysis by comparing peptide profiles from different experimental groups. Only this combination of different techniques and technologies allows the detection and identification of peptides as biomarkers by expanding common proteomic approaches into the mass range below 10 kDa.

Detailed and thoroughly planned and designed studies on the peptide content in correlation with defined pathologic states generate databases which combine information on physico-chemical properties of peptides with functional information against the background of a specific disease or condition, respectively. Such databases are the scaffolds for statistical analysis and data mining procedures such as network calculations and, finally, for biomarker discovery. The high number of analytes in combination with the biological variability and technical variation in sample collection and during analysis remains an extraordinary challenge demanding for high standards concerning reproducibility, throughput (sample number, group size) and dynamic range (quantification capabilities) of the analysis as a prerequisite for the performance of meaningful discovery studies.

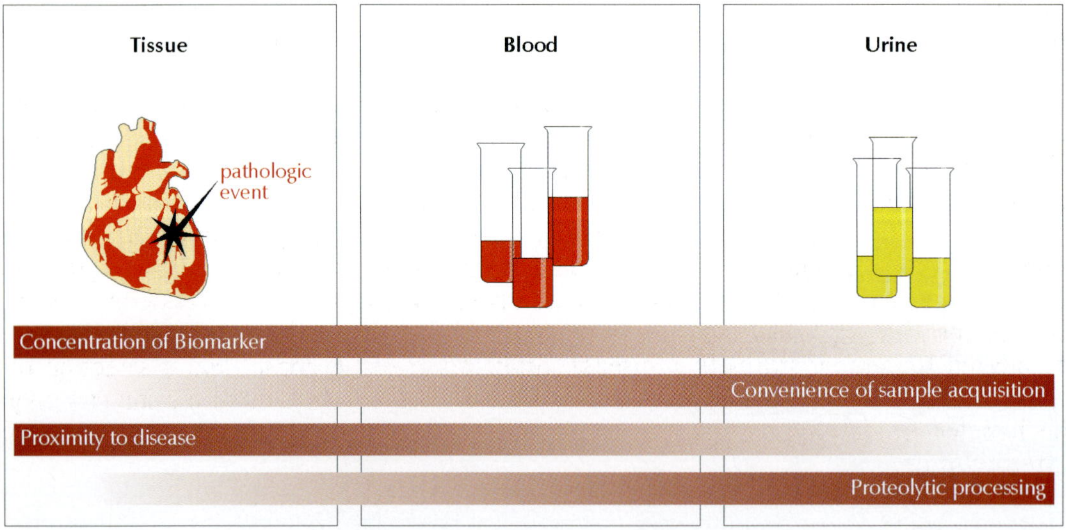

Fig. 10: Compartments of protein and peptide occurrence in the human body.
Protein and peptide biosynthesis, maturation and degradation takes place in different compartments of the body. The main human sample sources for discovery strategies are tissue, blood, and urine. The proximity to disease decreases in this order while the convenience of sample acquisition increases at the same time. In parallel, the concentration of a biomarker is diluted during its journey from tissue to blood to urine, accompanied by an increase in proteolytic degradation. Peptidomics studies focus on peptide biomarker concentrations, which are determined by sample availability, and the biological processes during secretion and diffusion.

Basis for such studies are a working hypothesis based on a possible involvement of peptides as well as the choice of the optimal sample matrix. The latter may result from a compromise between mere scientific considerations and the conditions in routine medical settings. Since peptides have the ability to traverse between compartments of an organism, many pathogenic processes are reflected by characteristic, pathognomonic changes of the composition of peptides in these body fluids. Peptides can be collected with these fluids in routine clinical settings and applied in diagnosis and therapy. Thus, the peptidomics approach in medical research is supported by the usually easier accessibility of extracellular human body fluids like blood plasma, urine, or cerebrospinal fluid as compared to disease-affected tissue samples. Nonetheless, in research projects it should be considered to target samples matrices which are as close as possible to the site of the primary pathological process (Fig. 10, see page 30).

In a compartment in the direct vicinity of a pathologic event the analytes' concentration is usually high with only a low probability of proteolytic processing. If specific differences are detected, it might be possible to correlate these data to the transcriptome, proteome, or peptidome of the affected tissue by analysing corresponding samples. During the process of biomarker detection and development it will be necessary to apply a variety of techniques to different sample types, shifting from a less specific screening method with blood to a more specific tool for the targeted analysis of previously defined tissue biomarker candidates in a compartment further down-stream. Urine is the endpoint source for many biomarkers, and the increased dilution or processing of a candidate has to be compensated by an increase of the analytical specificity and sensitivity.

In the beginning of a peptidomics discovery project, screening approaches bear the best chance of success. In case of peptide based studies, a comprehensive analysis of the peptidome delivers a plethora of information. Fig. 11 (see page 32) depicts some peptidomes generated from different types of samples. Small amounts of sample either from body fluids such as blood (i.e. plasma, serum, whole blood) or from tissues (liver, muscle, brain, tumour tissues) or cell cultures (supernatant, cell extracts) are sufficient to depict the respective peptidome of the sample. Specialised sample handling procedures need to be applied (or developed) depending on the high diversity of sample sources that may be used for peptide profiling. Separation techniques are required for the reduction of a sample's complexity followed by mass spectrometric analysis. In general, several thousand native peptides can be displayed, analysed for differential expression in relation to altered functional states (e.g. disease, drug treatment, exercise) and a selection of those will be transferred to sequence identification. This wealth of information can only be handled by specific software for multiplex analysis and skilled personnel for data interpretation.

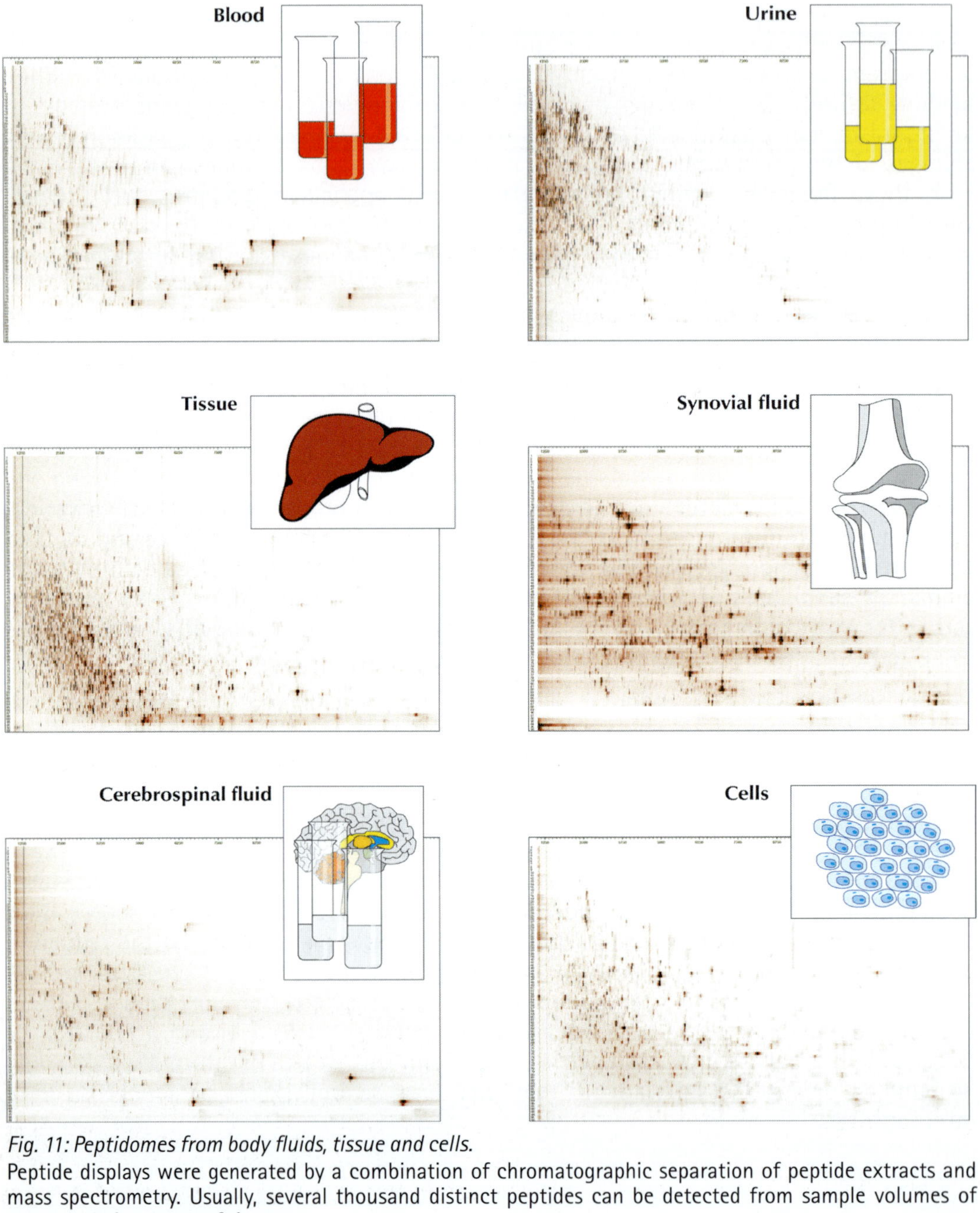

Fig. 11: Peptidomes from body fluids, tissue and cells.
Peptide displays were generated by a combination of chromatographic separation of peptide extracts and mass spectrometry. Usually, several thousand distinct peptides can be detected from sample volumes of approx. 1 mL or 1 mg of tissue.

1.6 Differential Peptide Display

Peter Schulz-Knappe, Hans-Dieter Zucht, and Michael Schrader

The concentration of peptides reflects certain information about the physiological status of an organism and this information can be uncovered using mass spectrometry for a comprehensive profiling of peptide patterns [1, 2]. Usually, peptide composition of any biological source is highly dynamic.

A detection system for peptides has therefore to fulfil two tasks in parallel: It has to show which peptides are present in a sample (qualitative analysis) and in what concentration (quantitative analysis). Only the combination of both will allow for the selection of those peptides that are valuable for the desired drug development process. We have named our way to analyse peptidomes in a qualitative and quantitative way "Differential Peptide Display". This strategy is *per se* not restricted to a specific type of analytical instrumentation, but we currently believe that a specific set-up allows for the best mix of resolution, sensitivity, throughput in terms of samples and sequence IDs, and quantification capabilities.

The MALDI time of flight mass spectrometer (MALDI-TOF-MS) [3] is a powerful tool for the comprehensive analytical profiling of peptides [1, 2, 4]. This instrument allows for the sensitive detection of peptide changes in complex mixtures of hundreds of different peptides simultaneously. Usually, a few micrograms of sample or cells are sufficient to create a detailed mass spectrum. The resolution and specificity of an analysis is further increased by coupling of mass spectrometers with liquid chromatography or other high resolution separation technologies. In our discovery cycle, the so called LC-MALDI platform is used (Fig. 12; see page 34) for peptidomics profiling. Here, biological samples are separated by means of high performance liquid chromatography (HPLC) into fractions and thereafter individually analysed in the (MALDI) mass spectrometer. The result of a peptide profiling process is a two-dimensional (2D) data set with the fraction number and a mass to charge ratio (m/z) as coordinates [2, 5, 6]. If proper care is taken with respect to reproducibility, sample preparation procedures and removal of excess proteins, the abundance of peptides is represented by the signal intensity in the mass spectra. This can be visualised in a two-dimensional intensity map using a color intensity code (Fig. 13; see page 35). Specialised software tools are used for data mining using such type of data for the discovery of differential peptide patterns. Usually, the differential analysis is complemented by means of statistical analysis for the exploration of the most significant changes in an experiment (Fig. 14; see page 35) [1, 2, 5-7].

In some approaches of peptidomics technologies, the separation step performed prior to MALDI mass spectrometry is kept simple resulting in a low resolution of the components but with considerably higher throughput at low costs. A typical example for a one-dimensional (1D) approach is the surface-enhanced laser desorption/ionisation (SELDI) platform. This technology is principally related to MALDI using a chemically modified chip surface to selectively capture and enrich peptides present in a sample for subsequent

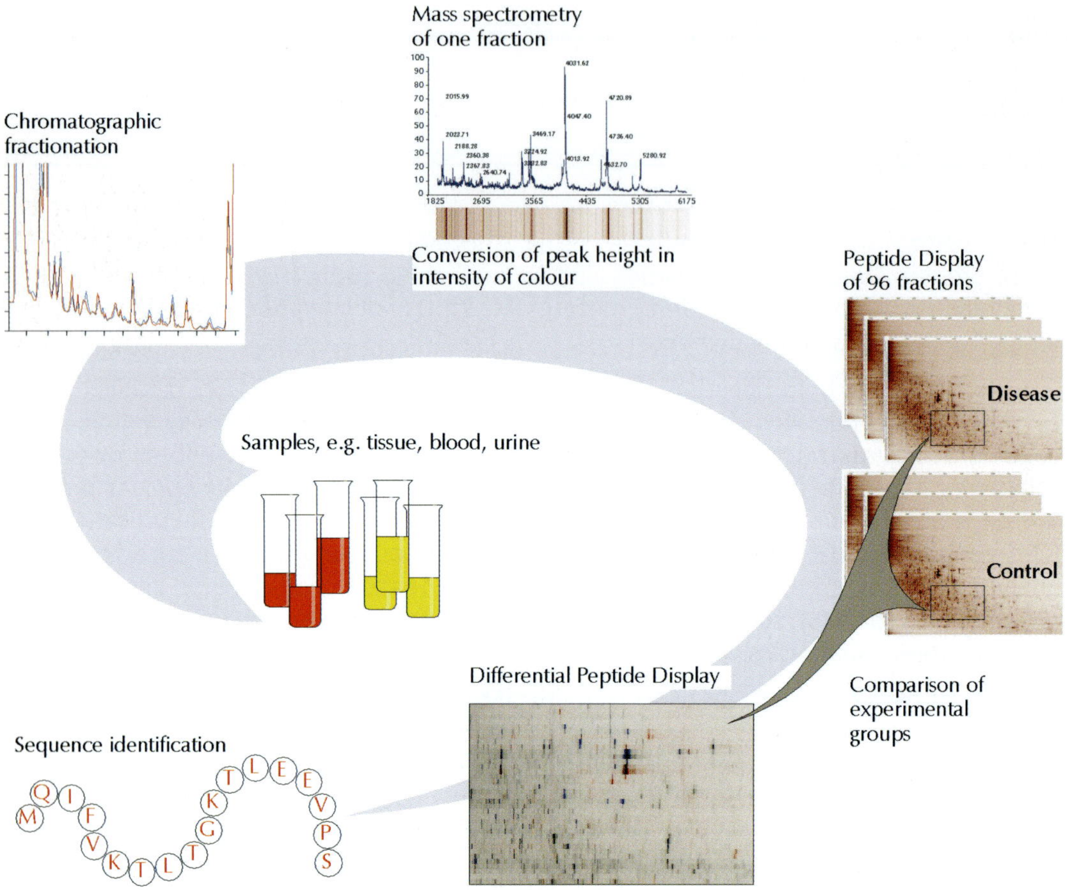

Fig. 12: Overview of the LC-MALDI based peptide profiling process.
Samples are chromatographically separated by means of HPLC. The fractions are subjected to mass spectrometry. The resulting mass spectra are depicted as 2D peptide displays and subjected to data mining procedures such as differential display analysis. Peptides that are differentially regulated are subsequently identified, either by MS/MS or Edman sequencing.

mass spectrometric analysis. Further technologies are currently evolving using magnetic beads or simple batch extraction steps for peptide extraction from body fluids [8, 9]. Both, the 2D and 1D approaches compare MALDI spectra fraction-by-fraction and exploit similar principles for data analysis [2, 6, 10–20].

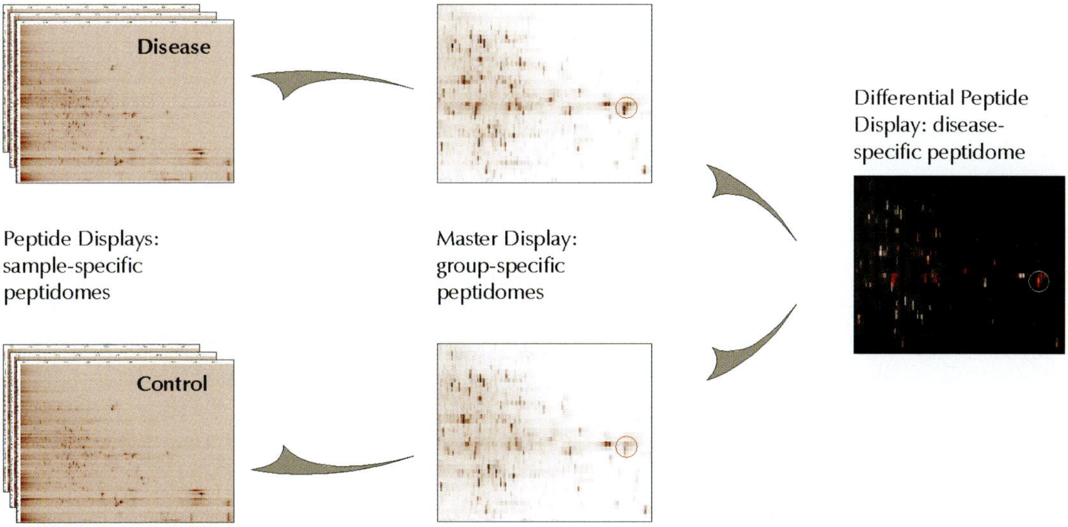

Fig. 13: Differential peptide display.

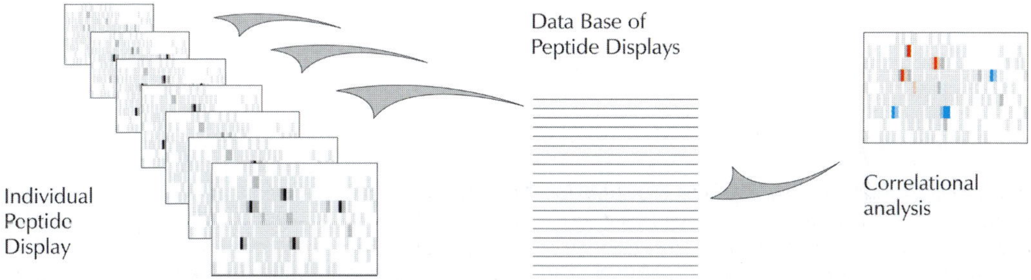

Fig. 14: Individual peptide displays are combined into a database for correlational analysis.

1.7 Bioinformatics and Data Mining

Hans-Dieter Zucht and Jens Lamerz

Mass spectrometry based profiling of peptides and proteins is used to distinguish groups of samples such as disease from non-disease and to monitor and predict drug effects. The combination of mass spectrometric with statistical analysis, yielding a general purpose diagnostic tool, has promising potential to enter clinical laboratories. Mass spectrometric experiments in peptidomics produce enormous amounts of data that raise numerous challenges in the fields of MS signal processing, statistics and experimental design. Data mining methodologies are required to support biomedical science, to manage these vast data sets and combine data from the measurement with other data from clinical settings. The workflow of peptide profiling, together with typical data mining methodologies will be outlined.

1.7.1 The MALDI mass spectrum

For the understanding of basic data structures, certain properties of MALDI TOF mass spectrometric technology need to be addressed. In the MALDI mass spectrometer, peptide ions are generated by laser excitation of the analyte/matrix crystals and accelerated to travel through a flight tube. They approach the ion detector at different time points that correspond to their specific mass to charge ratio (m/z), with low mass ions "travelling" through the flight tube at higher speed compared to higher mass ions, hence the name *time of flight spectrometry (TOF)* is used [3].

Peaks carry the relevant information of the mass spectrum. The shapes of peaks vary depending on the instrument's resolution, the change of peptide clusters during acceleration and flight, the peptides' nuclear composition and further characteristics of the device. This complexity makes the feature extraction a non-trivial challenge. The extraction of the intensity of peaks, which is related to a peptide's concentration, can be performed in different ways. For example, it is possible to use peak area measures after matching the peaks from different experiments. Alternatively, the intensity values of the histogram of certain bins can be used. Further data preprocessing steps such as binning, alignment of the spectra and intensity scaling to obtain a valuable data set are mandatory for increased data quality and comparability between sets of data, before data mining and statistical computations can be performed [21].

The measurement process has individual characteristics for each individual peptide. As a consequence, the characteristic dose-response curve differs from peptide to peptide resulting in a different sensitivity for any peptide. For example, the slope of the characteristic dose-response curve is related to the amino acid composition of the peptide and influenced by other peptides present in this same sample. It is important to mention that suppression effects in the measurement process can disturb peptide quantification. It should be carefully considered that the intensities of certain features

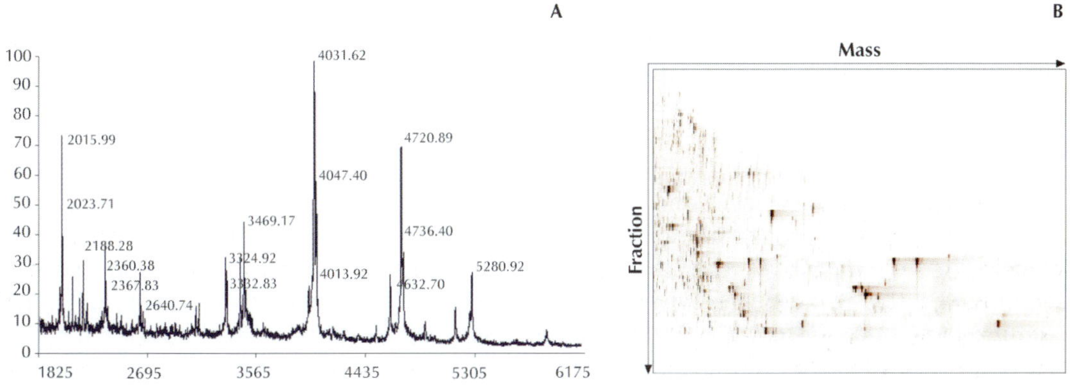

Fig. 15: 2D visualisation of LC-MALDI mass spectra.
A set of MALDI mass spectra (A) are assembled together in a data set referred to as peptide display (B). The mass spectrometric intensity is depicted in different colour intensities.

in one spectrum can be highly correlated with each other. A high correlation implicates that the features are not truly independent, which is important for certain statistical methods and for data interpretation. An important factor is usually the varying average mass spectrometric intensity. It is related to a general yield factor in the processing steps (pipeline effects) including sample preparation, peptide extraction, separation and mass spectrometric measurement. Further relationships are based on isotopic patterns due to the nuclear composition of peptides, signals from different charge states of a peptide, and signals caused by peptide disintegration. As a consequence, the result of data mining procedures has to be interpreted at the end with mass spectrometric expertise.

In a typical biomarker discovery study, samples from tissue or body fluids, such as human blood, are drawn from different persons or at different time points and analysed by mass spectrometry. The collection of mass spectra leads to large data tables, which are very general data structures providing a rich source of information. The dimensions of such tables are challenging: A typical experiment yields data structures containing over ten thousand features from every single sample, with a dimension of observations of a few hundred. The large number of features causes problems to establish generalized, broadly applicable models while avoiding the selection for patterns based on pure chance. There are different types of information that a scientist might want to extract from the data. He may not only wish to evaluate each feature separately, but may also be interested in patterns. Therefore it is necessary to apply statistics to extract as much relevant information as possible and reasonable.

The appropriate visualisation of MALDI mass spectra is important to understand basic structures in the data. For the visualisation of complex 2D LC-MALDI data sets, a two-dimensional map view has been introduced resembling the picture of 2D gel electrophoresis (Fig. 15). Such type of two-dimensional visualisation of statistical parameters provides a vivid interface for the data analyst.

1.7.2 Data mining

The term *data mining* is commonly used by statisticians and data analysts, while the term *knowledge discovery in databases* (KDD) is mostly used by artificial intelligence researchers [22]. Data mining is usually defined as the process of analysing data in a supervised or unsupervised, high-throughput manner to discover useful and relevant information that is hidden within complex data. The general aim of data mining is to answer three principal questions. The first question concerns the manner in which the objects, here the mass spectrometric samples, are related to each other. This is essentially a problem to cluster samples showing analogous peptide patterns. As an example, blood samples have to be correctly assigned to a disease or non-disease group, respectively. The next aim is to identify relationships between the features. Here, this means finding out which peptides are highly correlated with each other [7]. The final goal is the generation of models that describe the relationships between features and objects; these models are then applied for predictions or diagnoses. Usually, two modelling approaches are used in the medical application area. The feature-centric approach is aimed to find the most relevant feature, which is referred to as biomarker or diagnostic marker. In the focus of this approach are individual diagnostic markers providing a high modelling power. Such a marker should be compatible with existing medical theories and requires a validation of the novel biomarker with repeated measurements. The other approach exploits as many mass spectral features as required to provide as accurate predictions as possible. Black box models and marker patterns are capable of providing a high sensitivity and specificity during the predictions. However, the risk of overfitting models and a lack of a clear understanding about the underlying markers could result in limited acceptance in medical sciences, despite the fact that high public attention can be achieved. A validation of complex marker patterns is challenging.

1.7.3 First steps in data mining: projection methods

Projection methods are very helpful for the visualisation of highly dimensional data and for the grouping and extraction of the most important variables in a 'blind' unsupervised way in mass spectrometry data and for the identification of systematic errors.

One well-established method is the classical *principal component analysis* (PCA), where the information is represented by a new set of latent variables, termed components [23-25]. These factors are by definition orthogonal to each other and it appears that PCA is an adequate tool for the separation of principal phenomena that induce different variance. They could already give the answer to the primary analysis goal connecting it to a very global factor or they might even be related to unknown experimental factors.

There are some basic steps following any PCA analysis: after data collection and computation of the initial PCA solution, first principal components are, if possible, matched with appropriate interpretations, interpretation of the sign of the latent variables and finally analysis of the scores (e.g. relations of the samples) and loadings (e.g relations of the features) found. PCA is not well suited to pinpoint on individual feature properties because of its focus on global data structures. However, PCA is a powerful method if the biological question is related to the highest variance in the data set and for the purpose of outlier and process analysis.

1.7.4 Multiple statistical testing procedures

One of the most important methodologies for the analysis of relevant features in biomarker research are inferential statistical procedures, such as ANOVA, the analysis of variance [26]. The key method in ANOVA is the F-test that investigates the differences of means of a feature in two groups, e.g. one or several groups of the diseased subjects and the group of the control subjects. The t-test is a special case of one-way ANOVA with only two groups. Three parameters are reflected: the differences in means, group sample sizes and group variances. The parametric procedures in an ANOVA can be replaced by non-parametric procedures.

For data mining, such type of analysis is performed in a high-throughput fashion. The features have to be investigated individually and the p-values of each feature sorted top-down, to obtain the most relevant features in a type of interest list. This is essentially a design of multiple statistical testing, where thousands of hypotheses are tested simultaneously. The high number of features largely increases the chance of false positive results. For example, in an analysis of 10,000 features and not a single one is truly differentially regulated, one would expect $10.000 \cdot 0.01 = 100$ features to have a p-value equal to or less than 0.01. As a consequence, such experimental design needs an adjustment of the p-values or setting up a threshold for the prioritisation of the most relevant discoveries.

The investigation of the true distribution density function of the features is required for many statistical methods. However, the number of analysed samples, which is usually quite small, and the experimental set-up makes this task very challenging. As for any statistical set-up, power estimation helps to find out how many times an experiment has to be performed to avoid unrealistic expectations.

The most important method for investigating the role of individual features is based on correlation analysis – either parametric or non-parametric. It investigates a linear or continuous relationship between the features and a selected target variable. Such type of computation can even be performed with the data points of a whole mass spectrum. The results obtained can be visualised in form of a 2D peptide display (Fig. 16; see page 40). Usually, such types of analyses are performed in a similar way as described for ANOVA in a multiple testing design. For the selection of the most relevant features, the results can finally be sorted based on the (absolute) values of the correlation coefficients of the relevant features. Correlation analysis can also be performed to reveal relationships between the features themselves. Such type of analysis is done to create metabolic networks. This results in correlation associated networks (CAN) [7].

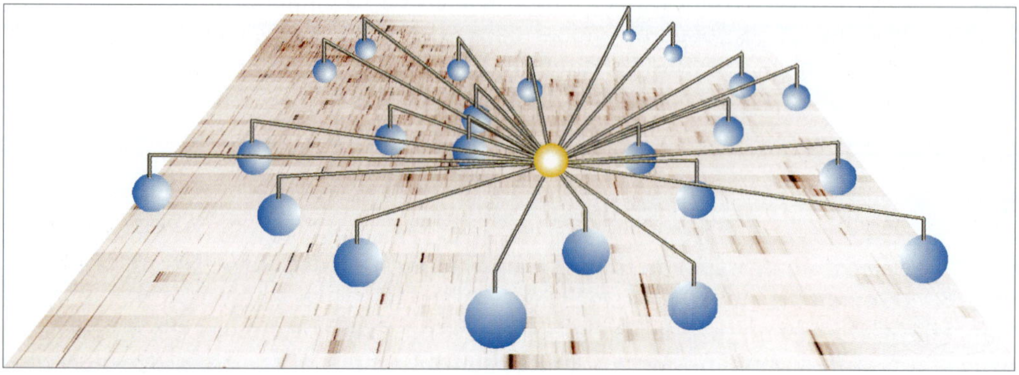

Fig. 16: 3D visualisation of a correlation associated network.
3D visualisation of a correlation associated network (CAN) of peptides (blue orbs) projected onto a peptide display. The network consists of peptides, whose concentration in independent samples correlates with the selected peptide (yellow orb) above a given threshold.

1.7.5 Outlook

Mass spectrometry gains importance for the analytical biochemistry especially in medical sciences. Two requirements drive the method developments: Medical research requires proper predictions of health conditions but also the ability of validating biomarkers and the predictive models for appropriate understanding. For the near future we expect an increase in sensitivity, dynamics and the resolution of mass spectrometers resulting in even larger data sets with a larger number of features. This will remain a challenge for data driven methods in the knowledge discovery process, which is a cycle of data driven and hypothesis driven work [27] (Fig. 17).

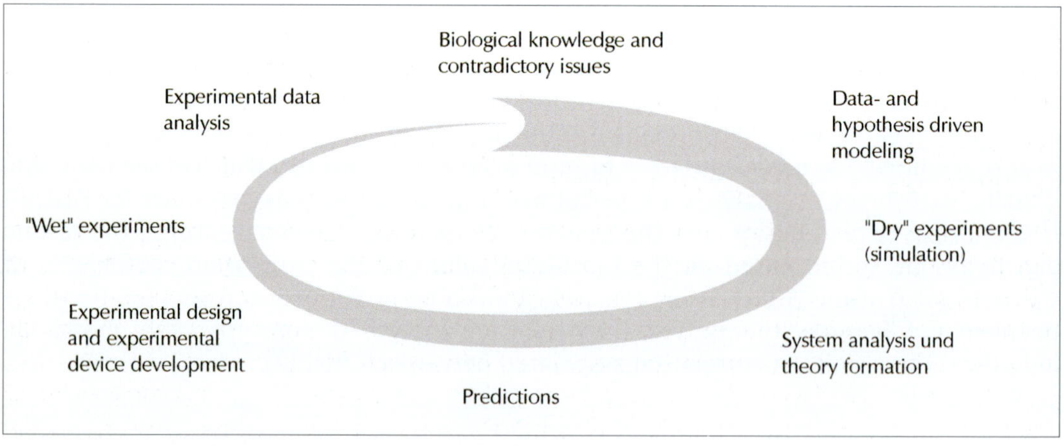

Fig. 17: Hypothesis driven research cycle in systems biology.

1.8 High-throughput Sequence Analysis

Markus Kellmann
and Christoph Menzel

1.8.1 Introduction

The term "sequence analysis" describes the revelation of the amino acid sequence of native peptides by instrumental and bioinformatic methods. In this respect, sequence analysis is considered as the indispensable link between the discovery process for biomarkers, usually by strategies such as differential peptide display, and the consecutive biological interpretation and validation of data. High sensitivity and specificity in sample discrimination can be achieved during a pure discovery process merely by the analysis of individual peaks or by pattern algorithms. However, without sequence information of the discriminating peptides, no in-depth information about the involved biological mechanisms or the pathobiological nature of the discrimination, respectively, is revealed. This will make any validation, reproduction of tests and standardisation for diagnostic applications a complicated task. Moreover, only a thorough sequence analysis avoids the risk of focusing on peaks derived from medium to highly abundant molecules, which may be of more general biological relevance. Examples are acute phase proteins or other abundant proteins secreted from liver which are likely to be involved in a wide range of diseases.

Sequence analysis for peptidomics can be performed either by mass spectrometric *de novo* sequencing assigning the full amino acid chain step by step "from scratch" or by identifying the peptide entity upon matching a characteristic mass spectrometric pattern of the sequence to a sequence database. With increasing coverage of (peptide) sequences in proteome or genome databases, the need for pure *de novo* sequencing is, however, decreasing. Moreover, for *de novo* sequencing a rather high data quality is required, since the full amino acid chain has to be unambiguously readable. In almost all cases, the faster and more widely used identification approach via a database match is therefore the method of choice for peptidomics purposes. As modern mass spectrometric methods outclass the classical Edman degradation microcharacterisation approach by orders of magnitude in sample requirement, sensitivity and speed, identification in peptidomics is nowadays almost exclusively performed by mass spectrometric methods. For confirmation purposes or in selected cases, Edman degradation will remain an option.

In the next abstract we want to detail upon important differences in peptide identification in peptidomics research compared to proteomics.

There, a whole industry has been built around the process to pick gel separated proteins, digest the gel pieces with trypsin and subject the usually 5-20 tryptic fragments to either peptide mass finger printing and/or MS/MS sequence identification. In contrast to this majority of identification approaches for proteomics, mass spectrometric peptide identification for peptidomics is carried out preferably by fragmenting the endogenous peptide entity directly (top-down approach) [28]. This means that no enzymatic or chemical digestion of the analyte molecule is performed prior to mass spectrometric analysis as carried out in conventional proteomics approaches. Although this "top-down" approach is technically more demanding, it has the clear advantage to maintain the full information on the polypeptide entity, which can get lost upon enzymatic cleavage. This is particularly the case if complex mixtures of endogenous peptides are targeted. As a consequence, only the endogenous analyte molecule itself is subjected to analysis and will give a MS/MS fragmentation pattern that is searched versus databases. The confidence-building analysis and matching of several tryptic fragments from one protein to the same database entry is therefore not possible.

Mass spectrometric sequence identification in peptidomics is performed by tandem mass spectrometry (MS/MS) [29]. Principally, a combination of two mass analysers is used in MS/MS. After ionizing the peptides of the fraction of interest via an appropriate ionization source, the first mass analyser selects a mass to charge ratio of choice (precursor m/z), followed by a specialised compartment of the instrument, typically a collision cell, breaking the precursor molecules into smaller fragments. The second mass analyser consecutively records the characteristic fragment masses. They can be matched against database entries for peptide identification [30].

For peptidomics research, two combinations of ionization sources and mass analysers are preferably used: MALDI tandem time-of-flight (TOF/TOF) MS/MS [31, 32] and nano Electrospray quadrupole-time-of-flight (qTOF) MS/MS [33, 34]. Differences as well as similarities of these both techniques will be outlined in the following sections on the basis of typical identification workflows that we developed for peptidomics. The data handling and bioinformatic processes to match the fragment ion patterns to a database entry are similar for all workflows, only adapting workflow or method specific parameters in the search algorithms.

1.8.2 Identification workflows

We distinguish three different workflows depending on the application area, the required speed and workload of the identification as well as the number and quality of peptides to be identified (Fig. 18, 19, 20; see pages 44, 46 and 47):

The first approach is the *overview* identification approach. The goal is a fast, cost-efficient, low material consuming but rather unspecific screening of prominent peptide landmarks using MALDI-TOF/TOF-MS/MS sequencing of peptides. In routine applications, we utilise the individual MALDI targets that were already used to produce the peptide displays for the biomarker discovery process. Precursor selection is performed randomly or in an automated mode using "on-the-fly" spectra evaluation software. Depending on complexity and average concentration of peptides, between 20 and 350 peptides per peptide display have been identified in projects from peptide displays that contained some 2000 peptides. This can be achieved from a single sample within a few hours in a fully automated fashion.

The second approach is the directed *biomarker candidate* identification, which consists of an in-depth sequence analysis of selected peptides, i.e. peptides with abundance differences as revealed in discovery studies such as differential peptide display. Here, after specific selection, only the peptides of interest are subjected to MS/MS experiments, using either MALDI-TOF/TOF-MS/MS or nanoESI-qTOF-MS/MS. In case of the MALDI-MS/MS experiments, individual peptide displays from the discovery process may be used as a sample source, especially since the metal target plates used for the initial MALDI analysis of individual samples can be archived. As soon as the biostatistical analysis of a peptidomics study reveals peptide biomarker candidates, the archived samples may be subjected to MALDI-MS/MS.

The complementary process utilises ESI-MS/MS experiments. Here, additional peptide material is required for sequence identification. Usually, remaining material from patients or controls is pooled and a peptide bank is generated as first step. A peptide bank consists of a semi-preparative preparation of 10- to 50-fold the sample material initially required for production of a peptide display. By use of larger HPLC columns and adaptation of gradient conditions, fractions that are very similar, if not identical, to the peptide display samples are generated and subjected to ESI-MS/MS experiments. Fractions are analysed manually or semi-automatically to achieve an unambiguous peptide identification for each compound. A biomarker candidate list typically covers 10 to 50 peptides, which can be identified within several days to weeks.

The third approach is the *inventory* identification approach which aims at a characterisation of a biological sample in a depth that is as complete as possible. To achieve this goal, a representative, semi-preparative or preparative peptide bank is created by repetitive fractionation of samples followed by subsequent pooling. Thus, sample heterogeneities are averaged and the sensitivity level for identification can be drastically improved. In our usual workflow, a peptide display of the peptide bank is generated that serves as the reference display of the biological source. Both MALDI and ESI based identification approaches are consecutively used to reveal the sequence of as many as possible peptides with corresponding peaks in the reference display. In case of the nanoESI-MS/MS technique, also a second chromatographic separation by means of an online HPLC-ESI-MS/MS coupling can be used to increase the coverage of identified peptides. An inventory identification typically covers hundreds to several thousand peptides from sources such as cerebrospinal fluid, urine, cancer cells or tissues. The corresponding analysis time for identification may span over weeks to months.

1.8.3 Overview identification

The overview identification approach represents the direct (online) high-throughput coupling of MALDI-TOF-MS based biomarker discovery and a first MALDI-TOF/TOF-MS/MS based identification (Fig. 18; see page 44). This allows the rapid identification of peptide identities in one instrument and from the same set of samples employing the same MALDI ionization source as in the MALDI-biomarker discovery process.

Selection of peptides for MALDI-MS/MS experiments is preferably based on MALDI-TOF measurements in the high mass accuracy reflectron mode. As outlined above, selection criteria for the overview approach are rather unspecific for the biological context, as the method is carried out independently of results from differential comparison.

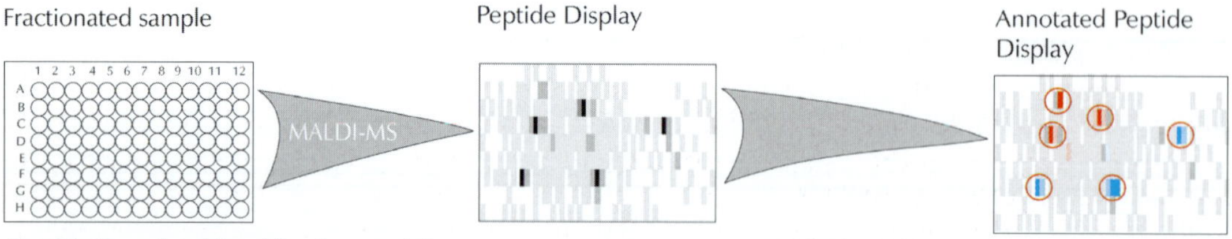

Fig. 18: Overview identification workflow.
Individual peptide displays from the biomarker discovery are subjected to a first unspecific sequence screening of prominent peptide landmarks using MALDI-MS/MS identification.

Typical selection parameters are therefore purely based on the mass spectrometric peak appearance such as a minimum signal-to-noise ratio or an upper mass limit. These selection criteria are chosen in order to contain peaks which have a higher likelihood to yield interpretable MS/MS spectra and, hence, are more likely to give a clear identification. Moreover, the selection criteria have to be accessible by the instrumental software in a fully unattended automatic fashion.

A particular limitation of the overview approach appears to be the accessible mass range for successful identifications. This is usually specific for the type of instrument used and lies in our MALDI-TOF-TOF-MS/MS based set-up currently at < 3.5 kDa. Nevertheless, this mass range covers an important, peptide-rich section of a peptidome. Moreover, several studies have shown that the overview approach is of particular value for quality assurance purposes or if a new sample source is analysed, as the accessible portion of the peptide display shows a good representation of sample specific features. Particular identifications representing deviations from the expected (source specific) composition are highly indicative and often allow for a first, biological interpretation of the whole sample set within the context of the study.

Among the deviations that most likely can occur analysing e.g. plasma samples are partial clotting of the sample and contamination deriving from cells such as erythrocytes (haemolysis), leukocytes and thrombocytes. Blood impurities in urine (post-renal affections, menstrual bleeding), cerebrospinal fluid (contamination during lumbar punctation) or in tissue biopsies are typical sampling artefacts, which can be traced down to the indicative molecular level in a timely manner. More generally, this also holds true for sample alterations such as oxidation or methylation of amino acids or the contamination from external sources such as from bacteria. Also, a rapid protease activity monitoring can be achieved by the overview approach, which is of particular interest in protease inhibition studies. Such a rapid monitoring might prevent wasting of a large number of precious samples from larger trials or wasting of analysis time on samples of poor quality. Moreover, every new sample source necessitates a thorough development of optimised peptide extraction and separation conditions. The rapid first order screening of the peptide content using the overview approach allows to guide the protocol development and accelerate it significantly.

1.8.4 Biomarker candidate identification

This process is insofar different from the "overview" process, as an underlying list of molecular masses from regulated peptides – generated from differential analysis of peptide displays from different disease states – is the starting point for peptide identification purposes. These peptides are well defined by their retention time (fraction) and molecular mass in the peptide display. The masses of these peptides range from 800 Da to 15 kDa. Due to the fact that the main components in the sample are regulated, but not disease specific, the bioinformatics output for disease specific potential biomarkers are commonly minor components in the peptide display.

The ideal case for identifying potential biomarkers is by means of an additional experiment from the identical sample. In the peptidomics process this is addressed by archivable sample targets, which are used for the discovery process as well as for subsequent MALDI-MS/MS experiments. Since the above mentioned limitations of MALDI-TOF/TOF-MS/MS and with respect to the minor components, "top-down" sequencing and sensitivity become issues. To perform "top-down" sequencing, the process is extended to a two-step process including MALDI-TOF/TOF-MS/MS and high resolution electrospray tandem mass spectrometry by means of a nanoESI-qQTOF-MS/MS instrument. The low sensitivity level is reached by generating an upscaled peptide bank for identification purposes only. This peptide bank, to be precise the peptide display of this bank (reference display), has to be most similar to the original peptide displays used for differential analysis to guarantee reliable cross annotation between those two displays. This is achieved by repetitive fractionating with subsequent pooling related to the same protocol used for preparation of the DPD samples. Typically, the sample amount is increased 5- to 10- to 50-fold compared to the discovery process.

After generating the reference display and locating the candidates on it, nanoESI-MS survey experiments will be performed on the desired fractions to locate candidates in the electrospray spectra. In our experience this is successful for approx. 80 to 90% of peptides, showing a rather high degree of concordance between MALDI- and electrospray MS output. NanoESI-MS/MS is then performed on the ions of interest with subsequent data reduction and database searching to identify them (Fig. 19; see page 46).

Combining the results of both approaches, the success rate of identification can reach 50 to 75% of the previous candidate list. The remaining 25% have to be identified by means of an additional chromatographic step with subsequent identification by nanoESI-MS/MS or Edman degradation or by manual or at least semiautomatic de novo sequencing. We want to state that there can be no guarantee that all peptides from an interest list will be successfully identified.

The candidate identification approach complements the differential peptide display discovery process and turns pure numbers in highly valuable potential biomarkers.

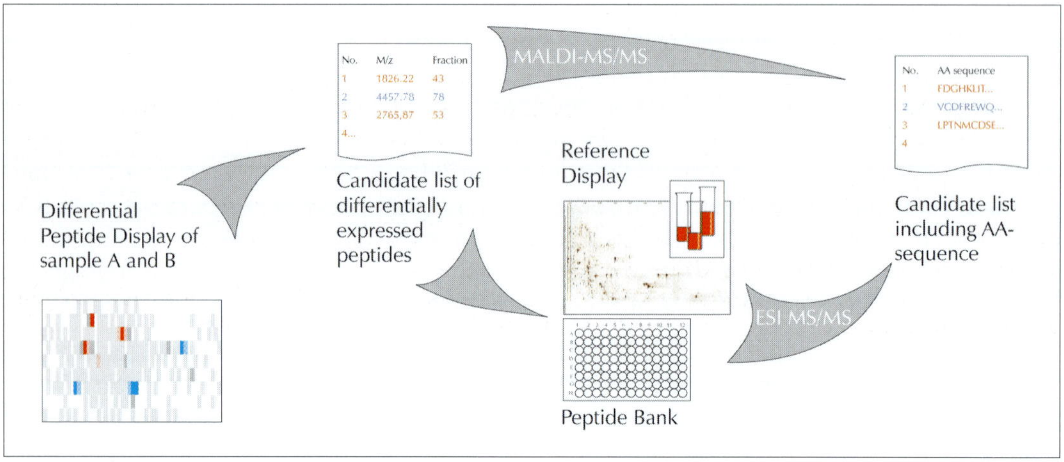

Fig. 19: Biomarker candidate identification workflow.
Candidate peptides, which revealed abundance differences in the DPD process, are subjected either to MALDI-MS/MS identification based on the archived display samples or to ESI-MS/MS identification based on separately generated reference samples.

1.8.5 Inventory identification

For some sample sources with high diagnostic value (e.g. human blood plasma, urine, cerebrospinal fluid) it makes sense to have a deeper view into the sample source than can be achieved by the overview approach and a more comprehensive approach than the DPD process can provide. This process is referred to as "peptide inventory" and aims at a detailed identification of about 50% to 75% of total displayed peptide signals. In the case of human blood plasma, the number of peptides to be identified is approximately between 1,000 and 2,000. Since this approach is also underlying a peptide display, namely the reference display of the sample source, the input in the process is not a candidate list from a differential analysis, but rather a list with signals from the reference display. This reference display is generated by MALDI-MS using a peptide bank, which is prepared according to the DPD protocol – but upscaled by pooling 10- to 50-fold sample amount compared to the amount applied to the DPD process. This procedure assures that all of the following steps can be carried out from one peptide bank referring to one reference display.

The generation of a peptide inventory normally starts with the identification of prominent landmarks. For this purpose an overview identification is performed by means of MALDI-TOF/TOF-MS/MS for the low molecular weight peptides up to a mass of 3.5 kDa complemented by a directed ESI-MS/MS analysis of unidentified prominent signals from

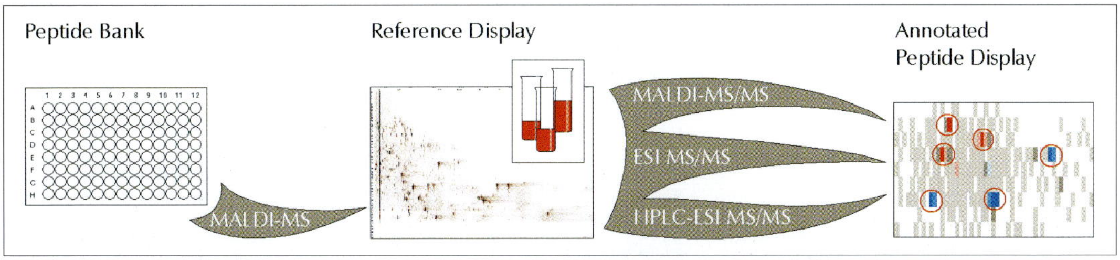

Fig. 20: Inventory identification workflow.
All peptide signals from a reference display are subjected to MALDI- and ESI-MS/MS (online and offline) identification for the comprehensive sequence characterisation of a biological specimen.

the MALDI-step and higher molecular weight peptides up to 10 kDa (Fig. 20). These two steps are directly performed using an appropriate aliquot of the peptide bank and yield 20% to 40% of the identifications. The remaining 60% to 80% can only be addressed by a further chromatographic step with subsequent MALDI-TOF/TOF-MS/MS or ESI-MS/MS identification, or in the case of peptides > 10 kDa by clean-up and Edman degradation. For the second dimensional chromatography, two or three neighboring fractions are pooled and submitted to another reversed-phase chromatography with different selectivity compared to the first reversed-phase step.

This "re-chromatography" can be performed online or offline to a mass spectrometer. The second dimension provides an additional decomplexification of the sample and concentration of single analytes, resulting in much higher identification efficiency. This step assures identification of minor components in the sample down to the pM range. Due to the fact that the creation of a peptide inventory is a matter of a mid- to high-throughput process (approx. 10,000-20,000 MS/MS spectra per inventory), it is required to automate hardware as well as software. For hardware automation, recently some helpful commercial solutions appeared on the market. For example, autoloaders for MALDI-MS/MS instruments and an autosampler for chip based nanospray are available. Both have been successfully integrated into the peptidomics identification routines to provide unattended MS/MS experiments where possible (Fig. 21; see page 48).

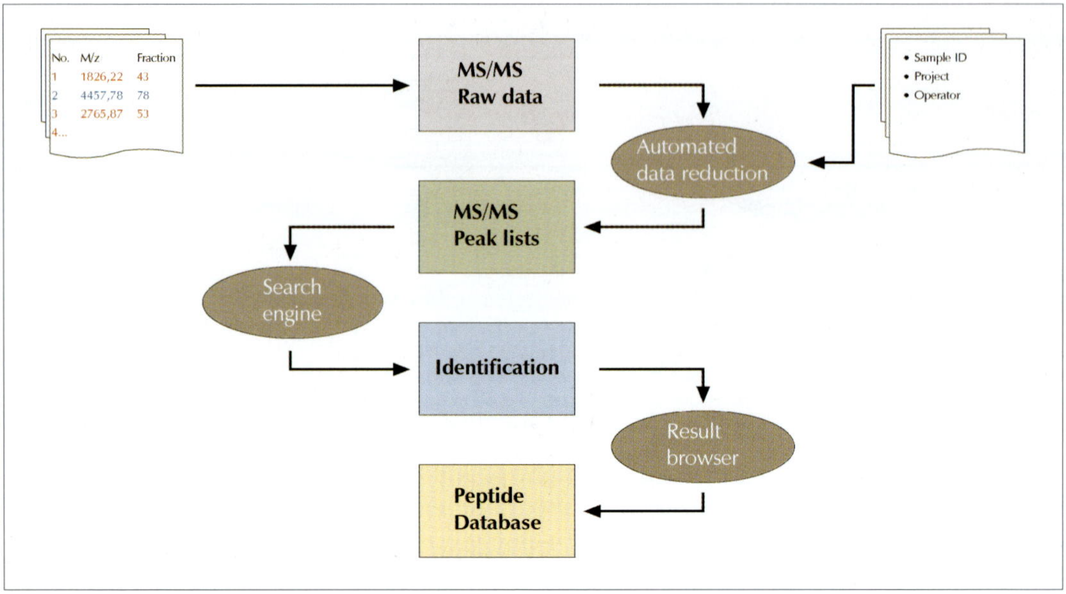

Fig. 21: General outline of the automated data flow in MS/MS experiments for the sequence determination in peptidomics.

1.8.6 Automation of data flow

Peptidomics peptide identification is a mid- to high-throughput process. To provide for smooth workflows, it is necessary to automate hardware *and* data flow and to link both. The heterogeneity of methods and instruments used and the high dynamics in the instrument market require a robust but most flexible data handling system. The complete data workflow for peptidomics sequence determination is shown in Fig 21. First, a so-called interest list (INPUT) is generated as described above. This list serves as the precursor list for any MS/MS experiment (either nESI-MS/MS or MALDI-MS/MS). After the MS/MS measurement, raw data from different manufacturers have to be processed and automatically searched against sequence databases.

For raw data processing, an instrument manufacturer independent data reduction tool is used, processing raw data from different vendors into peak lists ready to be used for database searching. Furthermore on this stage, sample associated data, such as sample source, project name, and identifier, operator and fraction position are included in the search file for complete sample tracking, before storage in the peptide database. The generated peak lists are searched automatically by the search engine steered by a remote client. Usually cascading searches including several databases (SwissProt, MSDB, IPI, dbEST) and multiple post-translational modifications (PTMs) are performed. The produced identification results will be filtered by a result browser and ranked according to their relevance. With this tool, ambiguous search results may be validated manually and included in or excluded from automatic import into the backend peptide database. This database is a relational database serving as a data warehouse for all generated peptide identifications, including amino acid sequence, PTMs, elution behaviour in the reference display (fraction), used instruments for identification, measurement errors, associated projects, sample preparation, literature and patent information.

1.8.7 Summary/outlook

The different identification approaches described here appear well suitable to address the different tasks in peptide sequence analysis for peptidomics. Of course, information from an overview or in-depth DPD-candidate experiment approach is not exclusive and can be used within one of the other workflows as well, similar to the methodology outlined for the inventory approach. The same holds true for the sequence information achieved by the different applied mass spectrometric techniques, which produce predominantly complementary information. Only the combination of MALDI and ESI ionization methods ensures a maximum coverage of positive identifications in peptidomics, in accordance to several proteomic studies comparing the identification power for tryptic peptides and both ionization techniques [35, 36]. From our experience in analysing lists of putative biomarker candidates with both methods, the more rapid MALDI technique is preferred for peptides smaller than 3 kDa, in particular for complex samples and samples with non-peptidic, low-molecular content contaminations that might affect electrospray ionization. With MALDI-TOF/TOF-MS/MS, those samples can often be analysed successfully, without the need to introduce additional sample clean-up steps or upfront-coupled LC chromatography. To also obtain peptide identification for larger native peptides, the nanoESI-qTOF-MS/MS is clearly recommended. In the overlapping mass range, where both techniques are applicable, the value of an affirmative identification should be exploited as much as possible to exclude any false positives before entering into subsequent biological interpretation and validation experiments.

Regarding the identification power, an increase in sensitivity and mass range width, particularly for MALDI-MS/MS, would be appreciated. Recently introduced derivatisation chemistries yielding higher fragmentation efficiencies might help to enhance the mass range for endogenous, native peptides [37, 38]. However, to achieve at least mid-throughput conditions, the introduction of robust, automated liquid handling for the derivatisation procedures is also required.

An alternative mass spectrometric technology with increasing popularity and excellent properties for the direct "top-down" identification of endogenous peptides and smaller proteins is Fourier transform ion cyclotron resonance mass spectrometry (FT-ICR-MS), especially when used in combination with electron capture dissociation [39]. Because of the very high resolving power of up to several hundred thousand and its excellent mass accuracy of a few or even less than 1 ppm, identifications of proteins up to 45 kDa have already been reported. Partly, low reliability and high acquisition costs and, hence, restricted availability are still limiting the routine application of this type of instruments for peptidomics purposes.

2 Applications of Peptidomics Technologies

2.1 Biomarker Discovery

Harald Tammen and Peter Schulz-Knappe

Biomarkers are important tools for basic and clinical research as well as diagnostic use. Different definitions of such a marker have been suggested, and all point out that it reflects the dynamic nature of physiological and pathological procedures in biologic systems. A widely accepted definition was worked out by the NIH Biomarker Definitions Working Group (1998) describing a biomarker as 'A characteristic that can be measured and evaluated as an indicator of normal biologic processes, pathologic processes or pharmacological responses to therapeutic intervention'.

In general, it can be differentiated between screening, prognostic, stratification and efficacy markers. Each type may be searched for and detected in tissues and extracellular fluids, i.e. body fluids in particular. The extracellular fluids represent the major link between cells, tissues and organs of an organism as a consequence of secretion, transport or diffusion and further processing of proteins and peptides. For all these different settings concerning purpose and localisation specific requirements regarding discovery and validation strategy have to be met, but the ability of marker quantification and identification are general key factors.

Several basic features apply for all successful proteomic and peptidomic biomarker research activities: Sensitivity, resolution as well as reproducibility of the discovery technology are crucial factors. Using a technology that fits the need of a biomarker discovery study, only samples of sufficient, i.e. usually high quality shall be included. The insufficient sample quality has been a common obstacle and sometimes even a reason for the failure of projects. It has to be pointed out that the term sample quality refers to specific requirements of the sample collection as well as the handling process that have to be precisely appropriate for the intended use. Unfortunately, we have to accept that there is no one "best way" to collect and store samples in a biobank, but that different sample specimens have to be collected from the same patient and stored in their specific, optimal fashion. This contributes significantly to the value of good sample material.

The initial step of a biomarker discovery programme will deliver marker candidates only. Specificity and sensitivity of such candidates have to be evaluated subsequently in defined and thoroughly selected patient populations. A comparison merely on the level of "diseased versus healthy status" is usually not sufficient. Different types and stages of disease should be included to allow for determination of specificity. In addition, a primary finding from a limited set of patients has to be validated in an adequate population of sufficient size and, taking the biological and environmental variability into account, in a multi-centre setting: It is well known that proteomes and peptidomes are highly susceptible in terms of biological and intra- and inter-individual variability, e.g. due to age, gender and nutrition. All this requires careful consideration when designing a biomarker discovery study for finding valid markers. Finally, a marker has to be matched with an available, and if possible, an accepted clinical endpoint as benchmark determined by independent analytical means, e.g. ELISA measurements [40].

Biomarkers hold great economical and medical potential, especially during the cost intensive drug development process. Monitoring of drug effects and efficacy by means of biomarkers will contribute to reduce the attrition rate of drugs during clinical phases and the overall development costs. For example, response and non-response to a drug may be characterised with the help of biomarkers and, therefore, only responders who will benefit from a therapy are included in clinical trials. Consequently, the concept of *"personalised medicine"* or the *"targeted treatment"* approach are dependent on the availability of appropriate biomarkers.

In contrast to the rising interest in biomarkers and the increased awareness of the opportunities following the application of biomarkers, less and less protein and peptide biomarkers/diagnostics are approved by regulatory authorities. One of the major causes might be the lack of adequate validation of potential biomarkers. Like compound selection for meeting pharmacokinetic criteria for a new drug, biomarkers should enable the same risk reduction for drug safety and efficacy. In the discovery phase, the high validation requirements for clinical access may often be underestimated. In this phase, efforts tend to be more technology driven, and the experimental design, especially sample number and selection, often lacks the long-term validation perspective.

In conclusion, a programme for the detection and establishing of a new biomarker generally comprises two phases, a discovery and a validation phase. The first one prospectively screens for new marker candidates that the second one seeks to confirm as suitable markers. In the screening phase a thorough planning and execution is of outmost importance addressing:

- hypothesis generation for any specific research scenario
- implementation of a suitable screening technology considering sensitivity, resolution and reproducibility
- definition of groups, e. g. disease or state of disease and corresponding controls
- selection of suitable samples (origin, collection, handling, preparation)

- sufficient statistical power/number of cases, i.e. samples
- tool for data handling and analysis
- techniques for disclosing the chemical nature of candidates in order to get insight in (patho-) mechanisms and to develop specific tests.

The subsequent validation phase concentrates on the confirmation of previously defined biomarker candidates by analysis of appropriate numbers of relevant samples using tools with a higher specificity and sensitivity than screening techniques.

Both phases together may deliver a biomarker or a pattern of several compounds that have proven against available benchmarks, preferably the existing gold standard, a potential to describe a physiologic or pathologic situation and indicate changes occurring under a challenge like a therapeutic intervention.

2.2 Biomarkers for CNS Diseases

Hartmut Selle,
Hans-Dieter Zucht, and
Martin U. Schuhmann

2.2.1 Introduction

A number of recent proteomics or peptidomics analyses in the field of brain research focus on cerebrospinal fluid (CSF) as specimen. Usually collected by lumbar puncture CSF is the adequate specimen for brain research. Though blood plasma might be considered as a more easily available analytical target it has to be taken into account that blood contains many proteins of extracerebral origin that may obscure Central Nervous System (CNS)-specific compounds. On the other hand the availability of brain tissue is limited in human research, thus CSF is the sample matrix closest to the place of CNS pathology. Though many compounds of CSF are of extracellular origin, a substantial portion originates from cerebral structures. CSF is generated by ultrafiltration of blood with a rate of 20 mL/h in the ventricles of the brain, from where it flows into the cranial subarachnoid spaces and subsequently the spinal subarachnoid spaces. About 150 mL CSF are constantly present in the cavities of the human CNS. It is absorbed back into the blood via the subarachnoid granulations and along the spinal nerve roots. Main functions of the CSF are the protection of CNS structures against physical impacts, the maintenance of a stable chemical environment, and the transport of soluble substances, especially the removal of brain metabolic products and the distribution of substances within the CNS, like electrolytes, glucose and immunoglobulins. On its way from the ventricles to the sites of reabsorption, CSF collects interstitial fluid from the brain tissue that is generated from the large surface of the blood-brain barrier and enriched by the extracellular components of the metabolism of brain cells. Therefore, CSF reflects both, CSF-brain barrier and blood-brain barrier function as well as brain cell metabolism, giving rise to the assumption that processes within the brain tissue leave traces in the CSF. Thus, CSF has been intensively analysed in order to obtain information from brain (patho-)metabolism.

It was introduced as diagnostic medium already in 1891: Frederiks and Koehler [41], Pearce [42] and Sakula [43] established the lumbar puncture and, in the same year, Toison and Lenoble [44] performed the first cell counts and cytologic examinations. Soon proteins were measured in the CSF [45, 46] establishing it as a part of clinical chemistry. In the 1940's, electrophoretic separations were introduced [47] which, in 1951, resulted in the establishment of CSF analysis by gel electrophoresis [48] which is still in use today. Beside the clinical examination CSF analysis was the most important neurologic diagnostic tool until the introduction of imaging techniques.

2.2.2 Collection of CSF

The lumbar puncture is an invasive intervention that is performed by specialised centres. Usually, no serious complications occur, but patients should rest for about 2 hours after puncture in order to minimise the risk of headaches. During the insertion of the needle a contamination with blood may occur and such samples should be strictly rejected since the comparison of specific compounds in independent samples of CSF and blood is an important diagnostic parameter (vide infra).

Though the sampling of CSF by lumbar puncture seems to be a relatively problem-free procedure, analytical errors in CSF analysis are caused by the heterogeneous situation within the intrathecal space. CSF composition within the ventricles and the spinal canal is quite different. The protein concentration in the ventricles is just half that of the lumbar concentration. Along the spinal cord, protein concentration shows a gradient. This led to the requirement to always collect identical volumes of CSF, which have to be collected at one batch before storing in aliquots.

Storage itself is more than just freezing [49]. Cells count should occur within the first 30 minutes as cells rapidly change their shape. Freezing has to be performed rapidly, cutting down the time at temperatures around the freezing point and at -11 °C, the recrystallisation temperature of ice. Since the immunoglobulins IgA and IgM show aggregation at low temperatures, a sample shall be kept for 30 minutes at body temperature after thawing to allow dissolving of such aggregates.

2.2.3 CSF analysis

With less than 4 lymphocytes per µL and only single monocytes normal CSF contains nearly no cellular structures. This facilitates the interpretation of analytical data revealing the occurrence of constituents of cellular origin (provided that a cell count is available for the specimen). Proteins are of specific importance in CSF based diagnosis of CNS disorders. Their content in CSF is increasing with age at about 35 µg/mL in adults. The protein content together with cell count and glucose content aid diagnosis and monitoring of disease progress of a variety of neurologic conditions, i.e. inflammatory as well as infectious diseases like meningitis, viral infections, and Lyme disease, demyelinating diseases (multiple sclerosis and Guillain-Barré syndrome), tumours of the brain and the spinal cord, cerebral and subarachnoidal haemorrhage. Microorganisms are identified from the CSF by staining, cultivation or immuno-based assays and agglutination tests. The ratio of albumin in the CSF and blood indicates the status of the blood-CSF barrier that may be impaired by infections, traumatic injuries, hepatic encephalitis or ischemia allowing an increased crossing of blood proteins into the CSF. During a blood-CSF barrier disruption, the CSF content of immunoglobulins also increases, but more important is the occurrence of IgG, IgA, and IgM which are synthesized in the CNS facilitating differential diagnosis of inflammatory diseases: IgG, showing an oligoclonal pattern in isoelectric focusing, is aiding the diagnosis of multiple sclerosis or early HIV encephalitis. Many bacterial infections like a cerebral abscess correlate with a significant local synthesis of IgA, whereas IgM synthesis is a characteristic of Lyme disease.

Although imaging techniques as well as the progress of neurosurgery revolutionised diagnostic access to the CNS, CSF analysis has moved back into focus for the quest of examining and understanding the function of brain proteins and especially regulative neuropeptides. Brain-born peptides not only mirror the processing and degradation of CNS proteins but they themselves may be specific bioactive factors that control a variety of physiologic and pathophysiologic processes. Therefore, the analysis of peptides in the CSF came into focus for depiction of processes within the CNS. Gel based screenings of the CSF revealed several hundred different cerebral polypeptides [50-52]. The mapping of a common pattern of CSF peptides, not only in single samples, in correlation with specific metabolic or pathologic events is subject to specific peptidomics technologies allowing a comprehensive peptide profiling of CSF samples, differential analysis of samples against the background of specific processes (differential peptide display), and pinning down differences in peptide patterns to concrete and identified peptides.

2.2.4 Peptide analysis for biomarker discovery in CSF

In a first attempt to systematically screen all CSF peptides in relation to a clinical condition, we analysed hundreds of CSF samples from patients with different underlying etiologies (Fig. 22). As an example, CSF was analysed from two patients suffering from primary CNS lymphoma (PCNSL). The resulting peptide pattern was compared with that obtained from the analysis of CSF from subjects without a CNS disease undergoing routine myelography. More than 6,000 signals were detected with a mass accuracy better than 500 ppm [5].

The precision of the chromatographic separation and the mass spectrometric analysis allowed the comparison of the two peptidomes. Several differences were found and a particularly distinct one was identified as a 24 amino acid fragment of serum albumin with the average relative mass of 2754 (amino acid residues 25–48). This peptide was detected with a higher intensity in samples from lymphoma patients than in controls (Fig. 23; see page 56). Only the identification of the peptide correlating to the mass spectrometric signal allows evaluating its pathophysiologic relevance. The increase of that particular albumin fragment can be explained by barrier disruption that typically occurs in tumour patients.

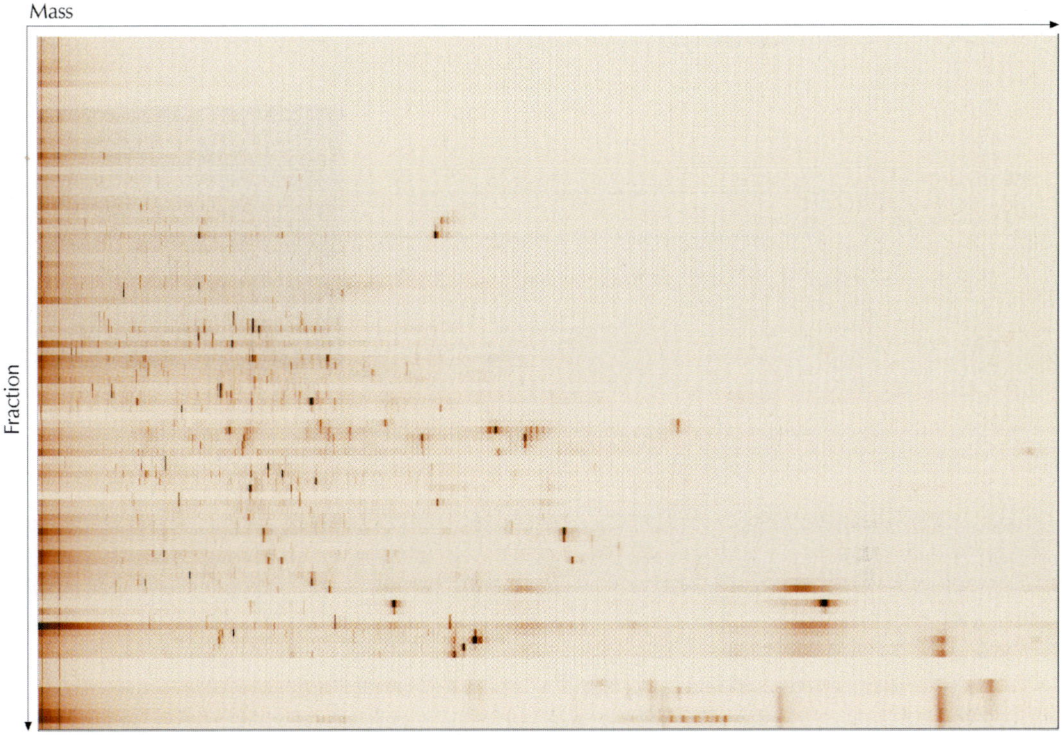

Fig. 22: Analysis of CSF by means of Peptidomics technology platform.

CSF samples were separated by reversed-phase chromatography in 96 fractions. Each fraction was analysed by MALDI-TOF MS (matrix-assisted laser desorption/ionisation time-of-flight mass spectrometry) and all spectra from one sample were combined to a multi-dimensional peptide mass display depicting the peptide pattern of the sample. For visualisation purposes, the intensity of each mass spectrometric signal is translated into colour intensity. Every bar represents a signal from the mass spectrometric analysis whose intensity correlates with the amount of a specific peptide in the sample. A typical display of CSF consists of more than 6,000 different signals, representing about 2,000 different peptide molecules with a molecular mass below 15 kDa. Each peptide's position is unambiguously characterised by its molecular mass and chromatographic behaviour, i.e. retention time.

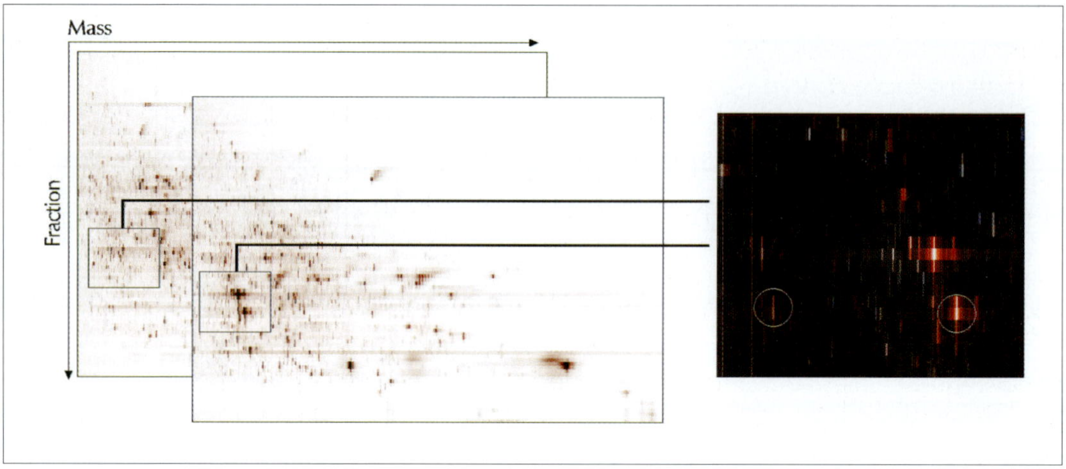

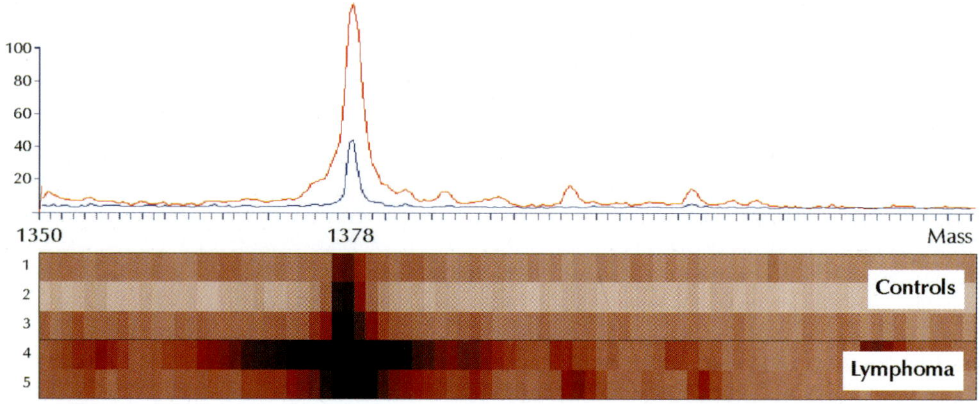

Fig. 23: Individual mass spectra generated from controls and lymphoma patients.
The signal of the double charged albumin fragment is depicted as the average mass spectrometric signal from lymphoma (red) and control (blue) patients (top panel). In the lower panel the spectra of every single CSF sample are given within a mass range between 1,350 and 1,450, after transformation of signal intensity into colour intensity. The signals from lymphoma samples are more intense, indicating that the corresponding peptide occurs in larger amounts in the CSF.

The complete albumin molecule is an established marker for the integrity of the blood-CSF barrier with the ratio of albumin concentration in CSF and blood correlating with the extent of the disruption [53, 54]. The smaller peptide might traverse the blood-CSF barrier more easily indicating a less severe barrier disruption at an earlier time point. Subsequent experiments with CSF samples from patients with different degrees of a barrier disruption (quantified by the albumin quotient of CSF and blood) confirmed the relationship between the intensity of this albumin fragment and the status of the blood-brain barrier. Therefore, CSF analyses should not only be based on comparison of peptide patterns but they should include also correlational analyses for establishing relations between candidate peptides and clinical parameters like the albumin quotient of CSF and blood. Another conclusion from this comparative experiment is that the differential peptide display of CSF allows a relative quantification of the peptide content by means of the mass spectrometric signal intensity.

2.2.5 Peptide analysis of rodent CSF

The differential peptide display technology has also been used for the analysis of CSF from rats. This experiment was, to the best of our knowledge, the first peptidomic study that addressed the complex situation of traumatic brain injury (TBI). Using the well established controlled cortical impact (CCI) model for induction of focal traumatic brain injury we analysed the change in peptide pattern within the first hours after injury as well as during a 7-day follow-up phase. More than 3,000 different peptide signals were screened and 8 distinct peptides were identified that showed significant post-traumatic changes. Neither these specific peptides, nor their precursor molecules have been specifically described in the context of TBI, however, their functionality was first gathered from literature in trauma related processes (publication Schuhmann et al. in preparation). This application of peptide analyses may be helpful not only for understanding trauma related changes in brain structures, their restoration and regeneration but also for the development of a neurochemical monitoring beyond the classical microdialysis parameters and of effective neuroprotective strategies.

In animal experiments not only CSF but also brain tissue is available for analysis. From rat hypothalami well-known neuropeptides were identified, demonstrating that peptidomics technologies are sensitive enough to even detect compounds in tissue that are of particular interest in brain research (Fig. 24; see page 58). Thus, well designed experiments with selected animal models may increase the chance to depict metabolic and pathologic processes in the brain by addressing the site where they occur and by analysing cell peptides.

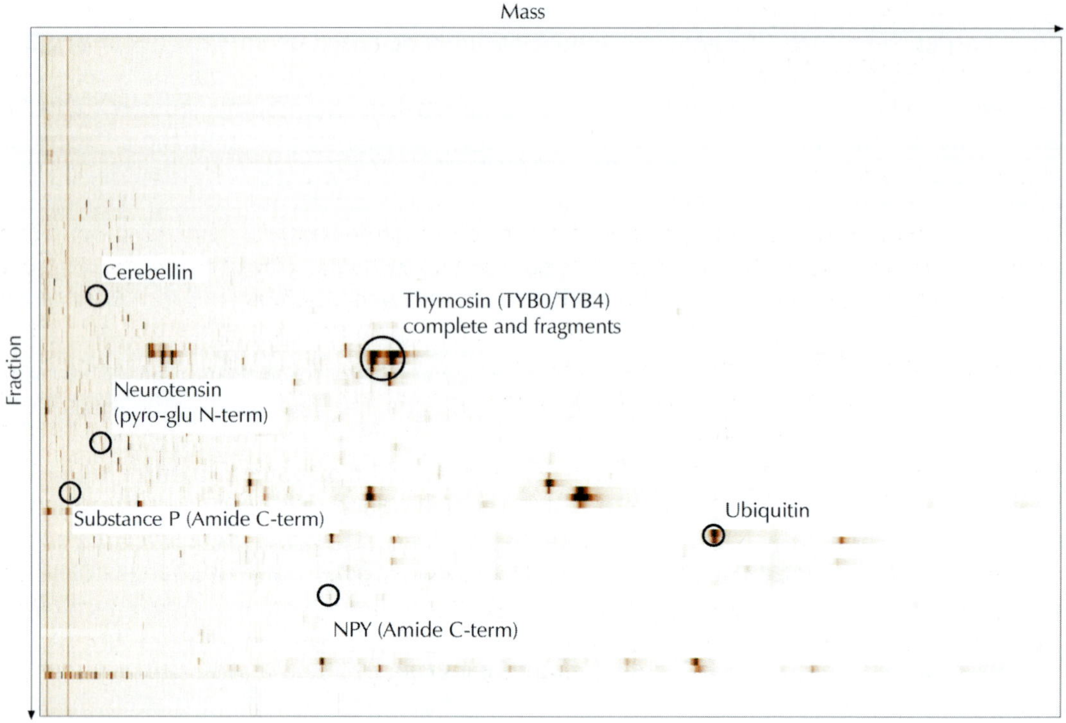

Fig. 24: Identification of peptides from brain tissue.
Rat hypothalami were used for the identification of brain related peptides. A range of peptides or fragments thereof were identified as indicated in the figure.

2.2.6 Summary and conclusion

The peptide screening of CSF is a highly suitable tool for the identification of biological markers that indicate significant events or conditions of the CNS, like the occurrence and the extent of damage to neurons or glial cells. Such markers can

- provide a deeper understanding of neurological and psychiatric disease by guiding research to pathophysiological mechanisms
- indicate disease related events that may allow diagnostic or prognostic statements or even reveal a new target for a therapeutic intervention.

The screening of proteins and peptides allows to identify patterns that may (i) depict more than one aspect of a pathomechanism, (ii) describe target pathways and (iii) cover all aspects of a therapeutic approach. Therefore we are confident that proteomics and peptidomics are relevant tools for the discovery of biomarkers for CNS diseases.

2.3 Analysis of Blood Plasma Peptides

Harald Tammen and Rüdiger Hess

2.3.1 Introduction

In the current activities on proteomics and peptidomics much emphasis has been given to the analysis of blood, since this source would by far offer the largest number of meaningful biomarker applications. The peptidome of a blood sample, frozen like a snapshot at the moment of blood withdrawal, throws light on the metabolic state of an individual. It represents a rich collection of information about physiological as well as pathophysiological processes occurring simultaneously. With this conceptual view, research in peptidomics follows concepts of in vitro diagnostics that rely on the assumption that a disease process in a tissue will leave its traces in blood. Therefore one clear aim of peptidomics analysis in blood is the detection of "the message from the tissue".

The blood proteome is considered to be the most diverse and might be the most challenging, though [55–57]. This is based on the fact that the majority of blood proteins, and presumably also of blood peptides, are from the liver. Some of these are present in amounts of several mg/mL, such as albumin, whereas biomarkers from other tissues are found in pg/mL amounts.

2.3.2 Specimen collection

Blood is a complex liquid tissue that contains a variety of cells and extracellular fluid, which are both utilised for analysis (Fig. 25; see page 60). Correct specimen collection is crucial to avoid or minimise artefactual processes (e.g. cell lysis, proteolysis) during specimen collection and preparation. To avoid coagulation, anticoagulants (mainly heparin, citrate or EDTA) are added into collection tubes, except when serum is needed. After blood withdrawal, ideally by a professional phlebotomist, the separation of cells and extracellular fluid is performed. To gently remove cells from extracellular fluid, centrifugation is routinely applied. Depending on the analysis technique used, this standard procedure is not always sufficient and further steps of centrifugation and/or filtration can be considered (Fig. 26; see page 61).

2.3.3 Protein depletion and peptide extraction

Analysis of plasma (or serum) on a proteomic display level is difficult due to the wide concentration range of proteins and peptides, spanning from millimolar concentrations (mg/mL) to sub-picomolar concentrations (pg/mL). The estimated number of individual peptides (blood plasma peptidome, also named low molecular weight (LMW) proteome, proteins $<$ 20 kDa) and proteins exceeds 100,000. Sample preparation for peptidomics aims to recover peptides and deplete or remove proteins. This is carried out by different physically (filtration) or chemically (precipitation) oriented methods commonly used,

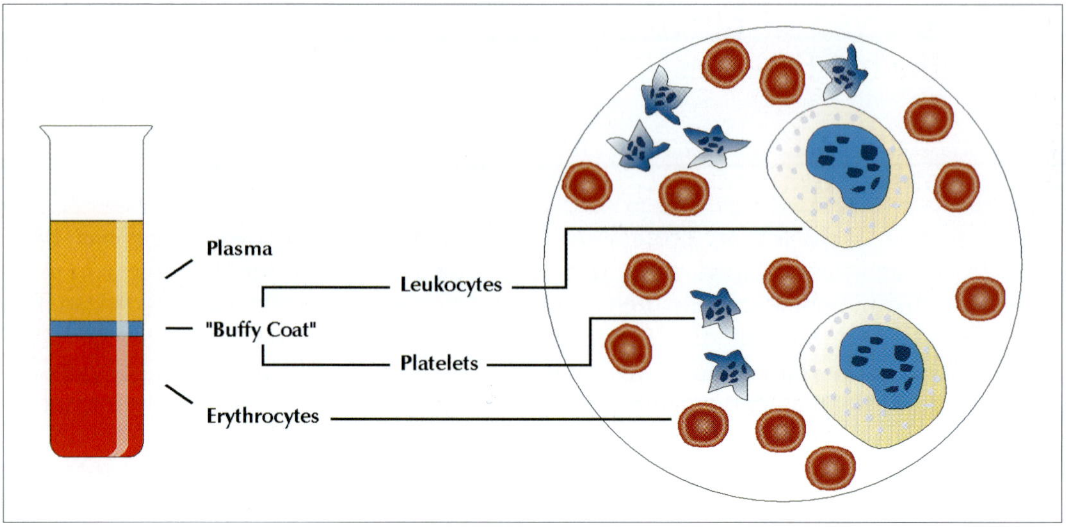

Fig. 25: Blood composition.
Blood can be regarded as a complex liquid tissue that comprises cells and extracellular fluid. For separation of the extracellular matrix (plasma) subsequent centrifugation steps can be applied. After centrifugation of blood three layers (plasma, buffy coat, erythrocytes) can be distinguished macroscopically.

which allow for the separation based on the molecular size. Also quite popular, immunodepletion of major abundant proteins can be performed. One important issue is to characterise the method for peptide extraction or protein depletion, respectively. Efficiency ("How many proteins remain in the sample after depletion?"), recovery ("What percentage of desired analytes is retrievable?") and reproducibility ("What is the coefficient of variation for the method?") are suitable parameters determined by immunoassays or protein assays.

HPLC fractionation and MS analysis

As outlined in previous chapters, the complexity of peptides in clinical samples is usually enormous. Therefore, peptide or protein extracts have to be prefractionated prior to mass spectrometry. This can be performed by LC (Liquid Chromatography) methods or on chip bound phases. After data generation, data analysis is possible by a plethora of data analysis tools, which are chosen depending on the purpose (e.g. detection/comparison vs. identification) and by integrating other relevant patient data into the analysis.

Applications of differential peptide display – determination of blood specimen qualities

Serum is widely used in clinical analysis, and many sample banks have large numbers of serum samples from clinical trials and epidemiological studies in stock. It is therefore important to analyse the usefulness of serum samples for proteomics and peptidomics studies.

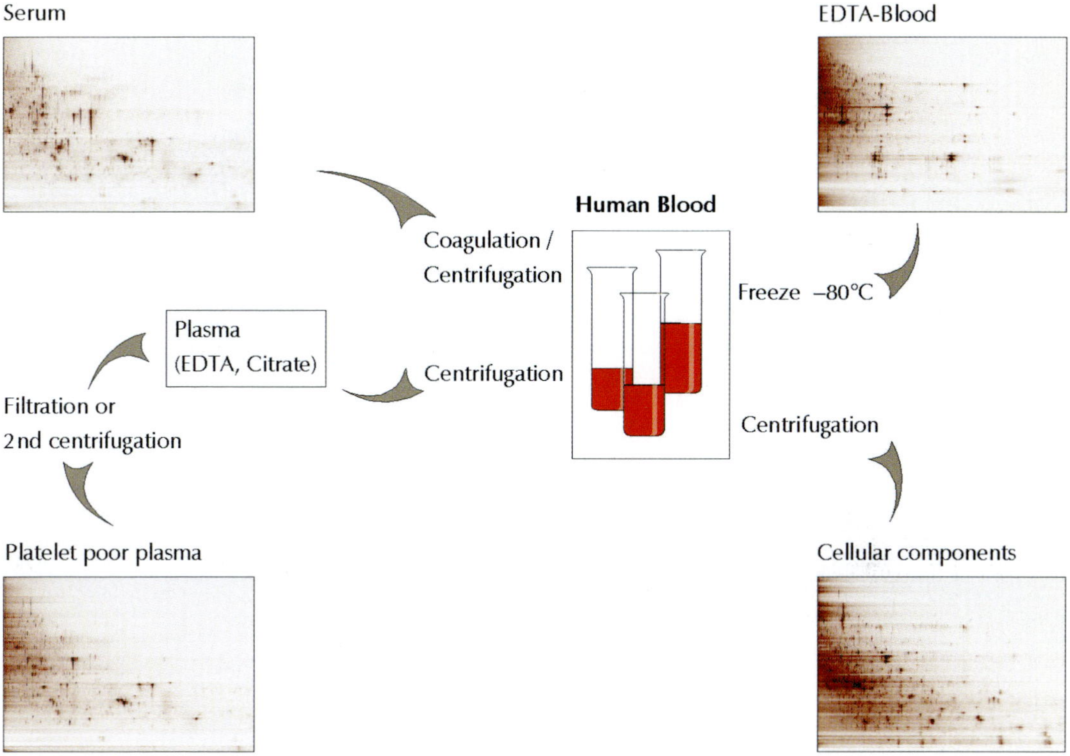

Fig. 26: Human blood specimens for peptidomics analysis.
After withdrawal of blood, various specimens are used for clinical diagnosis and research. Serum is generated by induction of clotting/coagulation; plasma is collected after centrifugation of EDTA or citrate containing devices and a second depletion step for platelets (sequential centrifugation or filtration). EDTA blood (whole blood) is frozen at –80 °C. Cellular components (e.g. platelets, red and white blood cells) can be obtained by centrifugation. Peptide displays of the various specimens are shown.

We performed an extensive peptide display study on plasma and serum samples, and compared the results in a differential display study. Comparisons demonstrate a high number of peptides which are only present in serum and not detectable in plasma, and many of them occur in serum in rather high abundance (Fig. 27; see page 62). This is in contrast to results comparing plasma and serum on 2D-PAGE where a high degree of concordance is given.

In fact, the high number of differences between the peptidomes of plasma and serum is no surprise, since clotting, which is only allowed in serum, is a multi-protease event with considerable power to assure effective coagulation. Consequently, many (highly abundant) proteins are cleaved by several proteases and thus release large quantities of peptides. These peptides are not seen on 2D-PAGE.

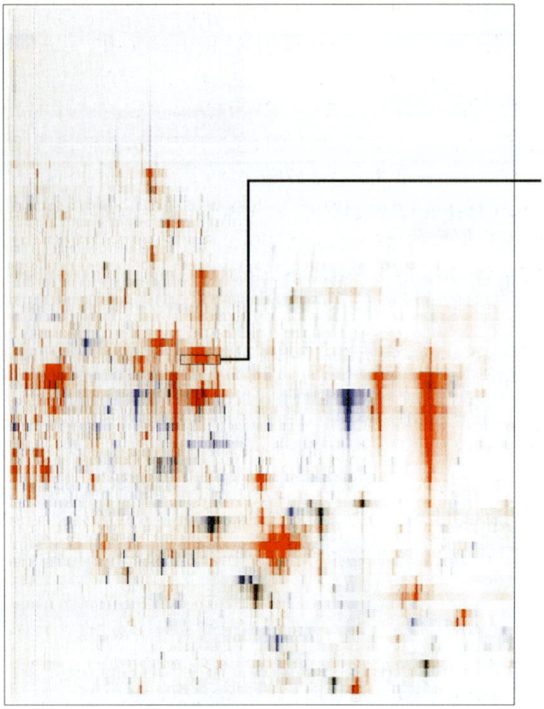

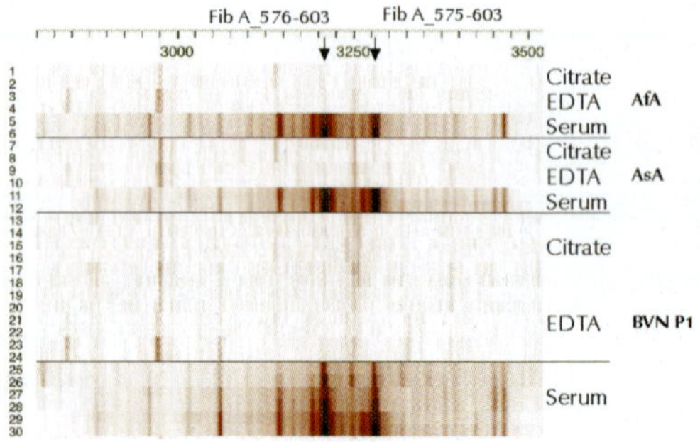

Serum Precursor	Cellular Origin
Apolipoprotein A-I precursor [Apo-AI]	
Collagen alpha 1[I] chain precursor	
Complement C3 precursor	
Complement C4 precursor	
Fibrinogen alpha/alpha-E chain precursor	
Fibrinogen beta chain precursor	
Myosin heavy chain, nonmuscle type A	+
Prothrombin precursor	
Serum albumin precursor	
Talin 1	+
Thymosin beta-4	+
Transgelin 2	+
Tubulin alpha-1 chain	+
Tubulin beta-1 chain	+
Vasodilator-stimulated phosphoprotein	+
Zyxin [Zyxin 2]	+

Fig. 27: Differential peptide display of plasma and serum specimens.
This heat map indicates differences between plasma (blue) and serum (red). Equal signal intensities are displayed as shades of gray. The upper inset depicts a zoom view into mass spectra representing a distinct chromatographic area and m/z region. 30 lanes from peptide displays (African American (AfA), Asian American (AsA), Caucasian (as representative example: BVN P1) of different specimens are shown. Fragments of fibrinogen alpha (arrows) are solely displayed in serum samples. The table depicts precursor proteins from peptides identified by MALDI-TOF-TOF in serum samples.

During the generation of serum from venous blood, various artificial processes occur that lead to ex vivo generation of peptides. With this term we refer to peptides that have not been present in vivo, but we want to emphasise that it may be possible that precisely these peptides may also result from in vivo processes. It is therefore important to verify whether peptides in a sample are a true reflection of the biology or a result from artificial processes.

After extensive sequence analysis of peptides that are highly increased in serum, these peptides can be separated into different groups. A significant number is derived from coagulation processes (like AP-FXIII; [58]), a further group results from other enzymatic activities (plasma kallikrein), and a third group reflects the release of peptides from the blood clot during specimen collection (thymosin beta 4, zyxin).

We conclude from our observations, that the use of serum for peptidomics studies is a complex task. In addition to the many artefacts that may occur, other factors influence the peptidome of serum. The composition of the resulting sample is dependent on several parameters such as temperature and time or medication of patients, which are hard to standardise in clinical routine or in cohorts. Furthermore, proteins may be bound to the clot, resulting in decrease of protein concentration during formation of the clot. In consideration of these data, serum shows many intense artificial peptide signals, which impede the sensitive detection of endogenous peptides. Nevertheless, serum could be helpful to validate results from biomarker studies, because it is the most archived sample in biobanks.

When plasma is generated in a conventional way, i.e. by centrifugation of EDTA blood for 10 to 15 min at 2,000 to 2,500 x g, red and white blood cells are sufficiently sedimented by centrifugal force without haemolysis. Upon close inspection, 20 to 50% of thrombocytes will still be present in the plasma. It is therefore recommended to remove residual platelets in order to obtain an optimal sample for peptidomics analysis. If platelets are left over in the plasma samples, a significant number of peptides from platelets will be detected in peptide displays. In addition, care has to be taken to avoid activation of platelets, such as cooling or agitation during sample handling (Fig. 28; see page 64).

As a further prerequisite for biomarker discovery, the peptide analysis technology has to be quantitative over at least two orders of magnitude. In a spiking study we could show that our dynamic range covers 3-4 orders of magnitude, depending on the individual nature of the peptide (Fig. 29; see page 65).

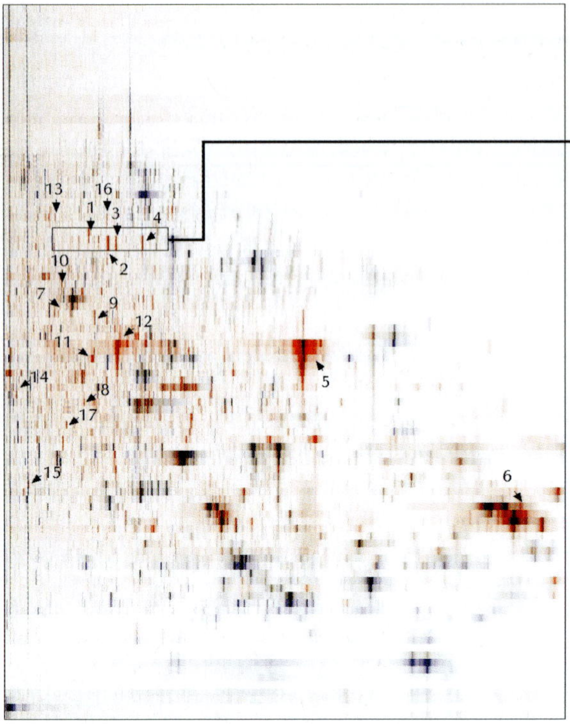

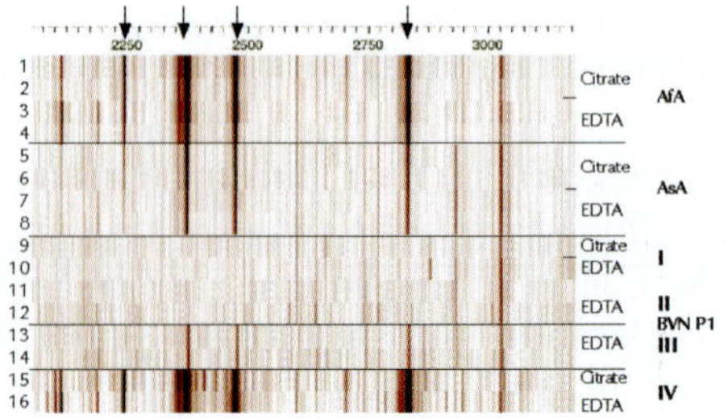

No.	Peptide	m/z observed	Swiss Prot Accession No.
1	TYB4_HUMAN 25-43	2113	PO1253
2	TYB4_HUMAN 23-43	2370	PO1253
3	TYB4_HUMAN 22-43	2471	PO1253
4	TYB4_HUMAN 19-43	2829	PO1253
5	TYB4_HUMAN 1-43	4963	PO1253
6	PLF4_HUMAN 32-101	7762	P02776
7	TBA8_HUMAN 358-373	1660	Q9NY65
8	TALI_HUMAN 449-466	1830	Q9Y490
9	ZYX_HUMAN 36-56	2188	Q15942
10	ZYX_HUMAN 20-35	1755	Q15942
11	TYB4_HUMAN 1-18	2151	PO1253
12	TYB4_HUMAN 1-21	2509	PO1253
13	TALI_HUMAN 434-448	1671	Q9Y490
14	TBA4_HUMAN 70-79	1184	PO1253
15	TBA4_HUMAN 260-270	1309	PO1253
16	VASP_HUMAN 281-301	2353	P50552
17	MYH9_HUMAN 2-16	1815	P35579

Fig. 28: Differential peptide display between plasma with residual platelets and platelet poor plasma.

This heat map indicates differences between plasma with residual platelets (red) and platelet poor plasma (blue) samples (EDTA and citrate). The upper inset depicts a zoom view into peptide displays representing a distinct chromatographic area and m/z region. 16 representative lanes from peptide displays (African American (AfA), Asian American (AsA), Caucasian (as representative example: BVN P1) are shown. Lanes 1-8: plasma with residual platelets, lanes 9-12: platelet poor plasma; lanes 13-16: Roman numerals refer to experimental conditions for plasma sampling: I: 2000 x g/RT/10 min/0.2 µm filter; II: 2000 x g/RT/10 min and 2500 x g/15 min/RT; III: 2000 x g/4°C/10 min and 2500 x g/4°C/15 min; IV: 2000 x g/4°C/7min and 1000 x g/4°C/5 min. Fragments of thymosin beta 4 are marked (arrows). The insert table lists the sequenced fragments of platelet associated peptides. The Arabic numerals refer to the marked peptides.

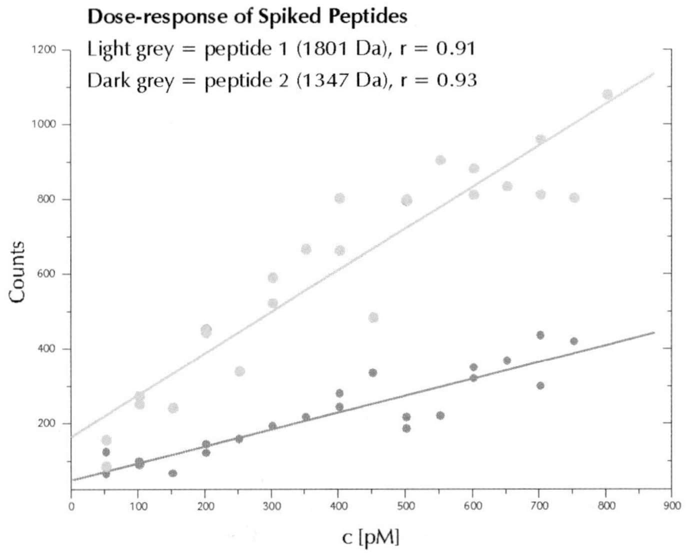

Fig. 29: Titration curves for renin substrate and substance P.
Different concentrations of renin substrate (1,801 Da) and substance P (1,347 Da) were spiked into blood plasma samples before processing. The resulting MS signal intensities are plotted against the spiked concentrations and show a linear dependency (light gray: renin substrate, r = 0.91; dark gray: substance P, r = 0.93).

2.4 Peptidomics Based Protease Inhibitor Profiling

Marco Jost, Petra Budde, Harald Tammen, and Peter Schulz-Knappe

Per definition, the proteome is the set of all proteins encoded by the genome and present in a specific time frame in an organism. While the genome remains stable to a large extent, the proteome is remarkably dynamic and different mechanisms of post-translational control exist. An important irreversible control level is proteolytic processing of proteins that releases an even larger number of peptides. Peptidomics concerns the characterisation of the full complement of small proteins and peptides in a specific organism, body fluid, tissue or cell type (Fig. 30; see page 66). Peptides are widely distributed mediators with roles in regulation of metabolism and cell function:

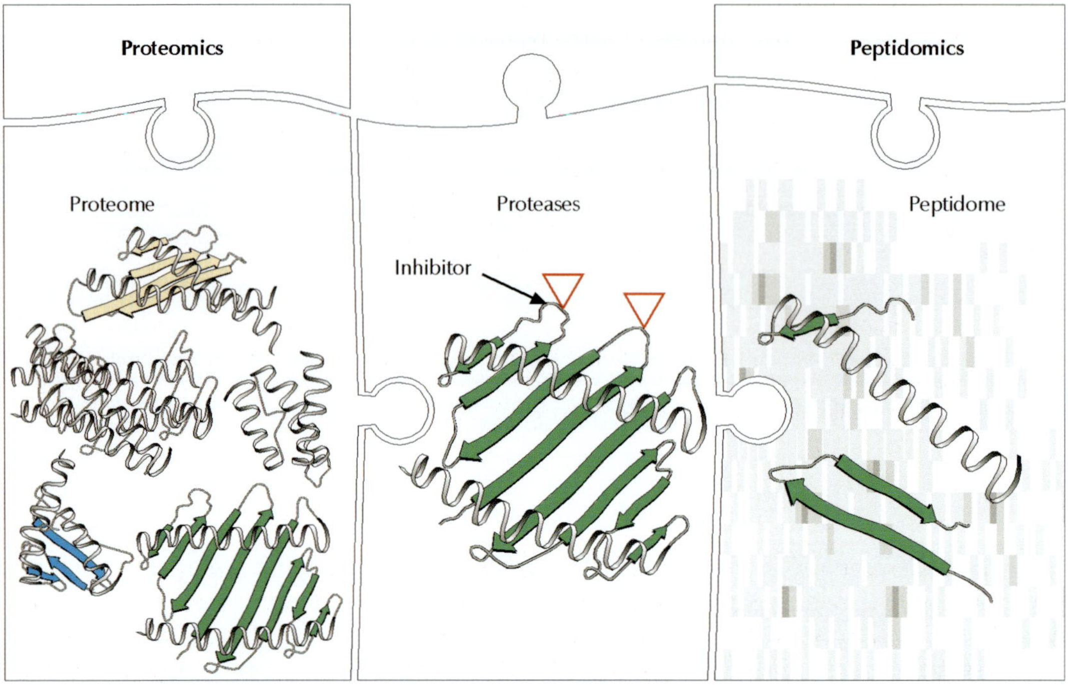

Fig. 30: The peptidome and the proteome are dynamically linked by proteases.

- Peptides act as hormonal messengers, cytokines, antimicrobial agents, and protease inhibitors. In the immune system peptides enable the detection of pathogens and viruses.
- The peptidome can be regarded as the metabolome of the proteome (Fig. 30). This makes peptides attractive to serve as biological markers of the physiological states and altered functions in diseased states.

2.4.1 The peptidome as an in situ library of protease substrates and products

Peptides are generated from larger precursors by the irreversible hydrolysis of a peptide bond. Because of this the peptidome reflects a natural library of proteolysis substrates and products. Proteases can be regarded as the signalling scissors of the body that initiate, modulate and terminate many important cellular functions by highly specific and limited substrate cleavage. An estimated number of 500 genes encoding proteases

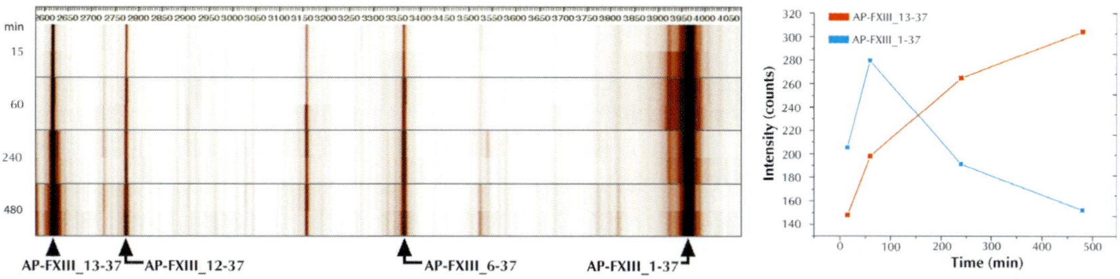

Fig. 31: Serum kinetics.
This panel depicts peptides generated by thrombin and plasma kallikrein during coagulation of serum samples in a time dependent manner (15 min to 8 hours). The graph illustrates the kinetics of degradation of the activation peptide of coagulation factor XIII (AP-FXIII).

and approximately 150 protease inhibitors have been identified in the human genome and many are of medical importance. Because of the success of established protease inhibitors targeting angiotensin converting enzyme (ACE) and HIV protease, proteases are increasingly viewed as valuable drug targets with application for the treatment of thrombosis (thrombin and factor X) and diabetes (dipeptidyl peptidase IV; DPPIV).

Current efforts to design therapeutic protease inhibitors are being accelerated by the increased availability of 3D structural information. Target protease structures are increasingly used to generate more selective, potent and better tolerated small molecule inhibitors. Approaches involve inhibitors that directly inhibit the active site or impair functions by binding to exo-sites and interfere with substrate or cofactor binding. To evaluate a protease as a potential drug target, it is important to identify its substrates and bioactive cleavage products. Detailed knowledge about protease substrates impacts the drug development process since specificity of inhibitors and thus limiting side effects can be predicted more accurately. Traditionally, the specificity of proteases is determined using standard or optimised peptide libraries containing small recognition sites or, for *de novo* screening, phage display libraries. However, protease inhibitor drug candidates are not exhaustively profiled against all other relevant proteases. Therefore, side effects may result from inhibition of the protease target or from a lack of inhibitor selectivity.

The peptidomics approach presented here aims to comprehensively profile the selectivity of an established protease inhibitor used in the management of thrombotic disease in an *in vivo* situation. It allows to identify protease substrates and products and complement the screening of inhibitor-library approaches to determine peptide-bond preference.

In initial experiments (see page 61ff. and Fig. 31), we observed pronounced differences between plasma and serum samples from the same individuals. Moreover, kinetic studies revealed that serum peptide displays changed drastically over time. This is an overall *in vitro* example for protease activity and kinetic analysis. The use of serum for peptide biomarker discovery is strongly affected by coagulation, but for specific cases the use of serum might be of advantage just because of this fact.

2.4.2 Coagulation

Venous and arterial thromboembolism represent a major health problem in the western world. Recently, a series of selective factor Xa inhibitors and direct factor IIa (thrombin) inhibitors have been developed and are close to broad clinical application. However, acceptance of new anticoagulants has been slower than expected because of the potential risk of more bleeding than with low molecular weight heparin. The challenge is to develop inhibitors with greatest efficacy but with the greatest degree of safety at a comparable cost. Comprehensive selectivity profiling of protease inhibitors in an in vivo situation should therefore contribute substantially to the success of future protease drugs.

According to the NIH "Hemostasis is induced by the activation of the coagulation cascade culminating in fibrin deposition through the action of thrombin on fibrinogen." The chief inducer of coagulation in vivo is Tissue Factor (TF), a 47 kDa glycoprotein. TF binds to factor VIIa, initiating a cascade of protease activation in which zymogen precursors are cleaved to their active form (denoted by the suffix "a") and resulting in the construction of prothombinase complexes (factors Xa/Va) on cell surfaces which activate thrombin (factor IIa; Fig. 32). The only cells capable of expressing TF in the bloodstream are endothelial cells and monocytes. By contrast, many cells outside the bloodstream, including adventitial fibroblasts, constitutively express TF and thus form an "extravascular envelope" capable of initiating coagulation in the event of a disruption in vascular integrity. The recognition of the central role of TF in the coagulation cascade has supplanted the classical notion of the extrinsic (or contact) and intrinsic pathways.

In addition to TF, platelets are critical both for the induction and formation of an adequate blood clot. Platelets act as a phospholipid surface upon which prothrombinase complexes are formed and act as a physical scaffold for the developing clot.

2.4.3 Counter-regulation of coagulation

The net procoagulant response represents a balance between processes initiating coagulation and those which inhibit coagulation or induce degradation of fibrin. There are three major anticoagulant and fibrinolytic mechanisms:

1. antithrombin III (ATIII), a serine protease inhibitor that covalently binds and inactivates active coagulation factors;
2. protein C, which is activated by endothelial thrombomodulin/Xa complexes and then degrades factors Va and VIIIa; and
3. plasmin, a direct fibrinolytic enzyme which is generated from its plasminogen precursor by secreted or cell associated plasminogen activators (Source: National Center for Biotechnology Information, http://www.ncbi.nlm.nih.gov).

To demonstrate the capability of peptidomics technologies to detect distinct changes in peptide profiles related to inhibiting specific steps in coagulation, a rat model for tissue factor induced disseminated intravascular coagulation was used to profile the synthetic

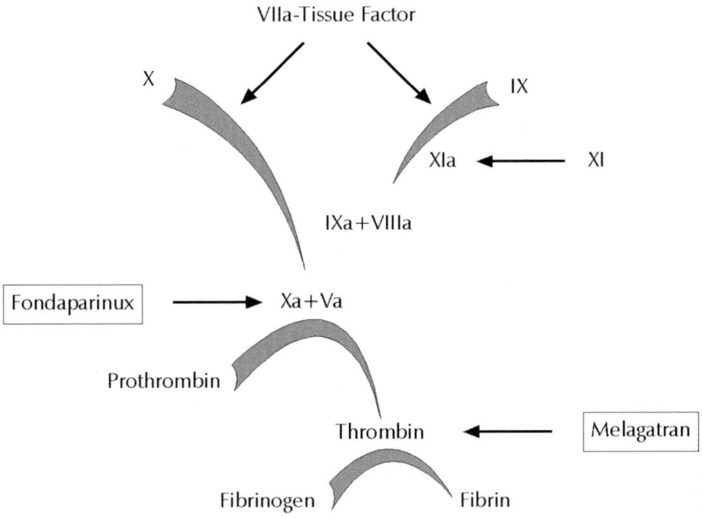

Fig. 32: Schematic representation of the coagulation cascade and sites of action of anticoagulant drugs.

pentasaccharideanalog Fondaparinux. Rats were treated with the tissue factor Thromborel S to activate the coagulation cascade in vivo. The degree of activation was monitored by determination of TAT (thrombin-antithrombin III complex). To modify the response, rats were also treated with Fondaparinux. Peptide displays were generated at baseline and after initiation of therapy. Comparison of peptide displays revealed differences in peptide abundance. Those peptides of interest were subsequently identified.

As expected, the sequence identities represent peptides that are directly involved in the coagulation cascade (e.g. fibrinopeptides or activation peptides).

The results presented here – using a model of intravascular coagulation in combination with peptidomics – provide a proof-of-concept for the integration of peptidomics studies into the drug development process. This study highlights the value of peptidomics in monitoring the effect of anticoagulating drugs in vivo.

2.4.4 Experimental design

Compound and tissue factor induced disseminated intravascular coagulation

Rats received Fondaparinux (Sanofi-Synthelabo) over a period of 2 hours via the *V. jugularis.* 1h after compound start, Thromborel S (Dade Behring) was infused for 1 hour. Blood samples were collected before compound infusion, 30 min after Thromborel S infusion, and at the end of Thromborel S infusion. The same experiment was performed with Thromborel S or Fondaparinux alone. For experimental setup see Fig. 33 on page 70.

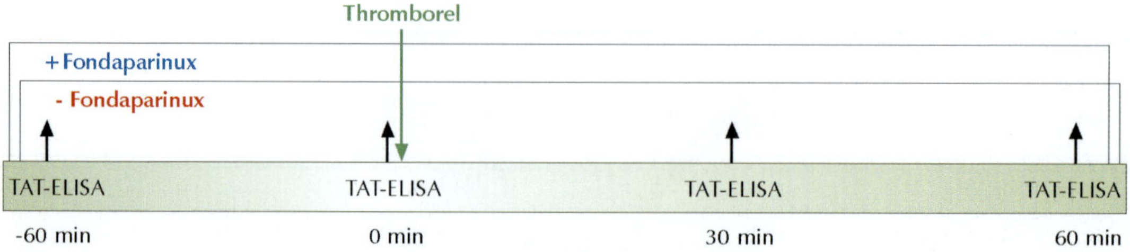

Fig. 33: Tissue factor induced disseminated intravascular coagulation in rats.
Rats received a bolus injection of 3 µmol/kg i.v. and a continuous infusion of 1.98 µmol/kg/h of Fondaparinux over a period of 2 hours via the right *V. jugularis*. 1 hour after compound start, Thromborel S was infused for 1 hour (7.5 ml/kg/h; prediluted 1:10 in 0.9% NaCl) via the left *V. jugularis*. Blood samples were collected in citrate containers (0.13 mol/l) before compound infusion, 30 min after Thromborel S infusion, and at the end of Thromborel S infusion via the left *A. carotis*. All blood samples were immediately centrifuged at 4°C for 15 min at 1500 g and stored at -20°C until determination of the thrombin-antithrombin complex (TAT) using ELISA.

2.4.5 Results

TAT levels were determined (Fig. 34) and peptide displays generated (Fig. 35). The TAT ELISA demonstrates the effect of Fondaparinux on FIIa generation. As expected, no changes were measured for aPTT. Anti-factor Xa activity was increased by Fondaparinux (>1.10 U/ml) compared to control samples (<0.01 U/ml) demonstrating bioactivity of the compound in the blood plasma following *in vivo* application.

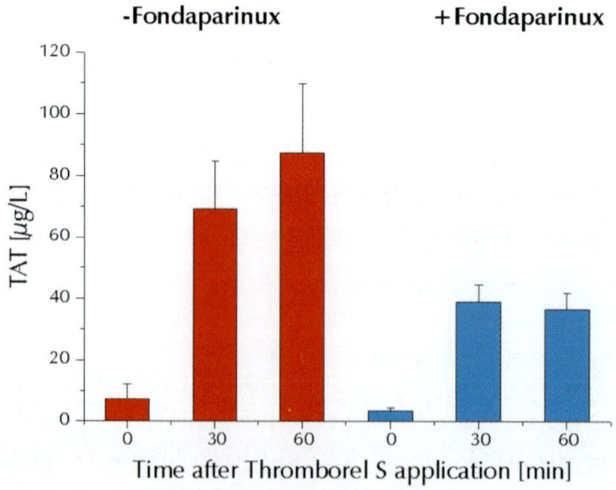

Fig. 34: Determination of TAT with thrombin-antithrombin ELISA.
Treatment with Fondaparinux (blue) leads to a reduction in the formation of the TAT complex compared to rats treated with vehicle (red).

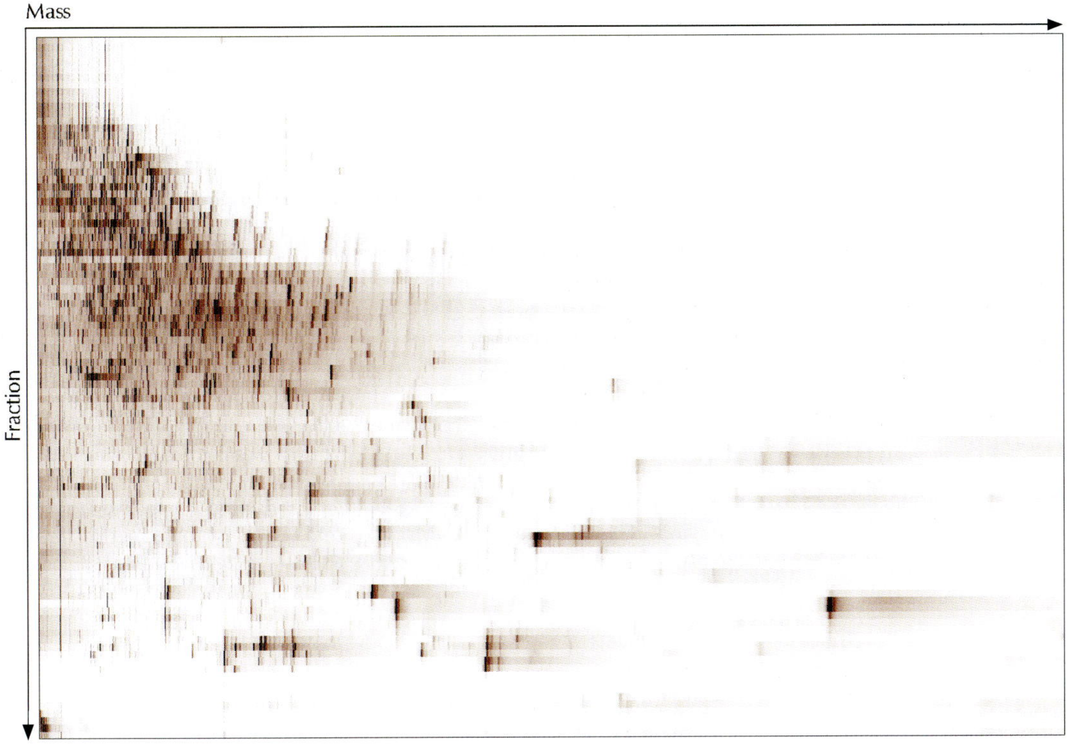

Fig. 35: Mean peptide display of plasma from animals treated with Thromborel S.

In all peptide displays, between 2000 and 6000 mass spectrometric signals are shown, corresponding to 1000–3000 individual peptides. This reflects redundancy (peptides that elute in more than one fraction), multiple-charge states, peptide species with and without oxidative states, and a small number of mass spectrometric derivatives, such as fragment ions.

Comparison of plasma displays from Thromborel S and Thromborel S/Fondaparinux treated animals reveal significant changes in the peptide pattern compared to controls (one example see Fig. 36 on page 72).

Four classes of peptide signals are detectable:

1. peptides that were not affected by the experiment;
2. peptides regulated by vehicle/Thromborel S and Thromborel S/Fondaparinux;
3. peptides regulated by vehicle/Thromborel S in comparison to controls and Thromborel S/Fondaparinux;
4. peptides regulated solely by Thromborel S/Fondaparinux in comparison to controls and vehicle/Thromborel S.

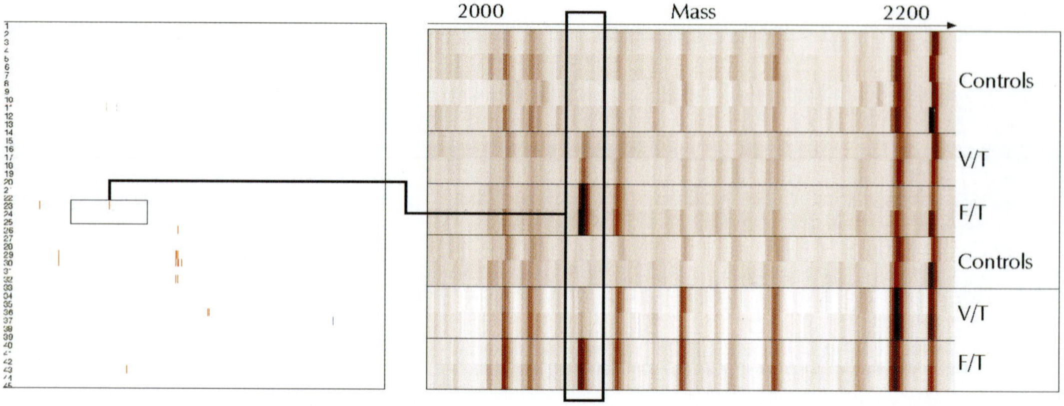

Fig. 36: Correlation display from Thromborel S/Fondaparinux treated animals.
Left: The correlation display depicts signals which are upregulated (red) or downregulated (blue) by Fondaparinux in comparison to controls and Thromborel treated animals.
Right: The graph depicts a zoom view into mass spectra representing a distinct chromatographic area and m/z region from peptide displays (controls, Thromborel S treated animals (V/T), Thromborel S/Fondaparinux treated animals (F/T)). A specific peptide (box) is upregulated in Fondaparinux/Thromborel S treated animals.

2.4.6 DPPIV inhibition

DPPIV (also known as CD26) is a multifunctional enzyme, acting on nutritional proteins, biological active peptides, and in immunological processes. DPPIV inhibitors are currently under investigation as a new class of antidiabetic drugs. Promising results have been obtained in preclinical and clinical studies showing the efficiency of DPPIV inhibiton to lower blood glucose levels. Drug action is mediated by preventing glucagon-like peptide (GLP-1) and gastric inhibitory peptide (GIP) degradation. These intestine-derived peptides, also kown as incretin hormones, are post-prandially secreted from enteroendocrine L- and K-cells and lead to a rise in insulin secretion. Several other peptides and proteins such as cytokines and collagens have been published to be substrates of DPP-IV. As the influence of DPPIV inhibition on these and possible other substrates and the corresponding in vivo effects are largely unknown, side effects may occur during chronic DPPIV inhibitor treatment. We therefore performed a study to evaluate the acute effect of DPPIV inhibition on blood peptides in a rodent model.

2.4.7 DPPIV inhibition induced effects on the blood plasma peptidome

Rats were treated with a DPPIV inhibitor or vehicle and blood plasma samples analysed by Peptidomics technologies aiming to identify distinctive as well as redundant alterations in the plasma peptide pattern. More than 3000 circulating peptides were shown in a mass range < 15 kDa. Additionally, DPPIV activity was determined in the same samples using GP-4 (glycine-proline-4) nitroanilide as substrate. At all tested concentrations (3; 10; 30 and 100 mg/kg body weight) a maximal inhibition of ~88 % of the DPPIV activity was reached (Fig. 37 upper right panel). Differential peptide display reveals signals which are decreased or increased following treatment with the DPPIV inhibitor.

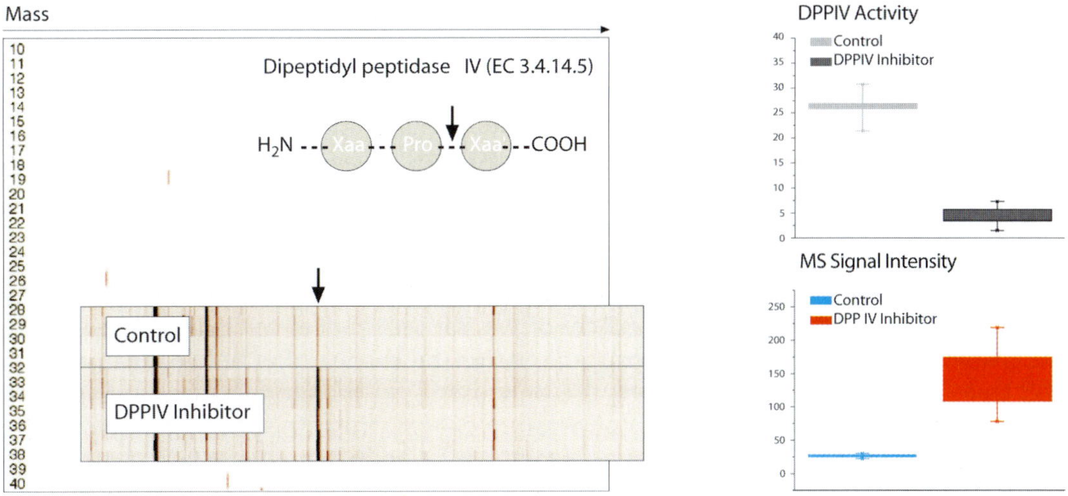

Fig. 37: In vivo inhibition of DPPIV.

Rats were treated with DPPIV inhibitor or vehicle and blood collected after 6 hours by cardiac puncture. Plasma peptide displays were generated and correlated with their respective DPPIV activity. The resulting correlation display depicts peptides with are positively (red) or negatively (blue) correlated with the inhibition of DPPIV. Using this approach signals were identified which show an increase in MS signal intensity (black arrow) in multiple samples whereas DPPIV activity is reduced as graphed in the upper box-and whisker plots. These signals were identified as DPPIV substrates by their N-terminal cleavage motif as depicted in the inserted sketch.

Peptides with increased abundance retained the N-terminal consensus DPPIV cleavage motif (Xaa-Pro-Xaa) and are suspected substrates for DPPIV (Fig. 37). In contrast, peptides which are abolished by DPPIV inhibition are putative products of DPPIV action (as detected in controls without addition of inhibitors) and are further degraded by other blood plasma proteases (e.g. degradation by plasma kallikrein).

2.4.8 Conclusion

A plethora of changes occur in blood peptide composition in vivo during protease inhibitor treatment. These changes and their alteration by drugs can be observed in experimental settings by differential peptide display. Using a factor Xa specific inhibitor, peptides with proven involvement in the clotting cascade were identified to be differentially regulated (e.g. fibrinopeptide A; protein C). Additionally, testing the effect of DPPIV inhibitors in vivo revealed the accumulation of substrates containing the DPPIV cleavage motif. The protease inhibitor specificity profiles analysed provide a "fingerprint" of the inhibitor action in vivo. Unlike other currently used methods to determine inhibitor specificity, peptidomics screens comprehensively all peptides altered in situ upon inhibitor treatment irrespective of pre-postulated optimal substrates. This information will be useful for dissecting physiological pathways affected by protease inhibition and can be applied to monitor drug activity and specificity in vivo. The identification of putative biomarkers in this setting can be further used to improve the development process of novel protease inhibitors.

2.5 Cancer Biomarkers

Harald Tammen

A key application for all "omics" technologies is oncology. A plethora of new drugs are under development, most of them based on insights in molecular biology, and a growing number of biomarker applications exists. This is because primary prevention is not feasible for most cancers, and cancer pathogenesis is not yet well understood. In the past 20 years the survival rates of patients with advanced solid carcinomas improved only modestly. The 5-year survival rate of cancer patients shows a high correlation to tumour stage. Therefore, early detection of cancer offers the best chance for cure. Consequently, the axiom of "the earlier the diagnosis, the better the chance of effective treatment" is still true. Today most tumour markers are only useful for monitoring therapy. Even one of the most useful tumour markers for prostate cancer, prostate specific antigen (PSA), is of limited applicability due to its non specific elevation in benign prostatic hyperplasia (BPH). Therefore, discovery of a biomarker for early detection of cancer is one main goal in cancer research.

2.5.1 Peptidic tumour markers

In the recent years proteomic techniques evolved, which offer new perspectives in discovery of new cancer biomarkers based on the detection of low molecular weight (LMW) proteins (peptides) by mass spectrometry. Peptides are especially promising tumour marker candidates for several reasons:

1. In contrast to proteins peptides are more capable of reflecting pathological aberration due to stochastically increased probabilities in peptide processing.
2. Peptides are smaller than proteins; therefore the possibility to migrate between different compartments is higher and hence the chance to detect peptides apart from origin of the disease is increased.
3. Peptides are not as well evaluated in terms of biomarker suitability as proteins.

A tumour marker is a substance present in, or produced by a tumour itself, or produced by the host in response to a tumour. It is used to differentiate a tumour from normal tissue or to determine the presence of a tumour based on the measurement in blood or other fluids. Morphologically cancer tissue is recognised to resemble fetal tissue more than adult differentiated tissue. In general, many tumour markers represent the re-expression of substances normally produced by embryogenic tissue (e.g. AFP, CEA).

The development of a new cancer biomarker consists of a discovery phase and a validation phase. The discovery phase aims at finding putative candidates for further validation. On this note the validation phase summarises methods for determining the predictive value of a biomarker and not the validity of the test system used for discovery.

The number of candidates derived from the discovery phase should be limited because the validation of too many candidates exceeds a feasible validation design. Therefore it is essential to design the discovery phase in such a way that only the most promising candidates are selected for further validation. To establish a valid tumour marker the issues of specificity and sensitivity have to be addressed. A marker should be produced by the tumour cell and be detectable in body fluids. It should not be present under healthy or benign conditions. To generate a tumour marker panel with sufficient specificity special attention has to be paid to selection of tumour stages and control groups.

2.5.2 Oncopeptidomics

Two main peptidomic approaches for tumour biomarker discovery are currently under investigation: pattern recognition vs. single/oligo biomarker detection. In 2002, Petricoin et al. [126] published results about the usage of SELDI-TOF-MS for mass spectrometric pattern acquisition from serum samples of patients with ovarian carcinoma and control groups and the application of bioinformatics tools (e.g. genetic algorithms) to separate cancer from controls with high specificity and sensitivity based on MS patterns. Major concerns addressed by the scientific community (especially E. Diamandis [56]) were

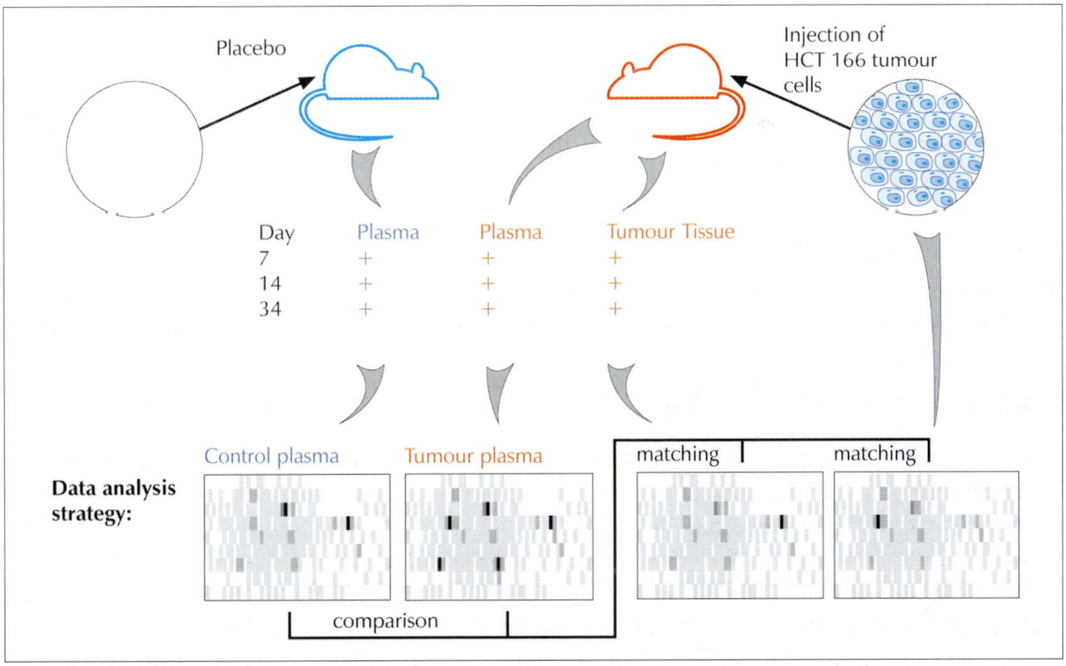

Fig. 38: Experimental design.
SCID mice received HCT 116 xenotransplant or placebo. At different time points, plasma and tissue samples were collected and analysed by DPD. Additionally, peptide displays from cell culture supernatant and cell extracts were generated.

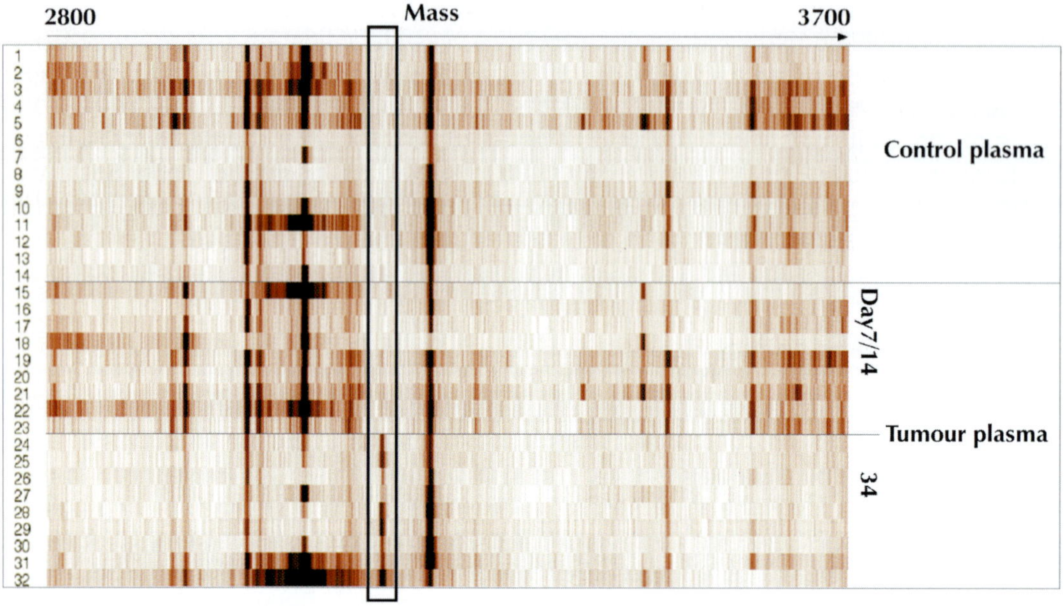

Fig. 39: Detection of differences.
The graph depicts a zoom view into mass spectra representing a distinct chromatographic area and m/z region. Thirty-two lanes from peptide displays (controls and tumour bearing mice at different time points) are shown. Human Tif-1ß (box) is present exclusively in tumour bearing mice plasma samples

- the lack of sequences and consequently a biological hypothesis,
- the questionable choice of control groups,
- the discrepancy between sensitivity of SELDI-MS compared to concentration of hitherto known cancer biomarkers,
- bioinformatorical overfitting of MS data.

Until now a distinctive conclusion can not be made and large studies are currently in progress to reveal the benefit of MS pattern based cancer diagnosis (NCI, EDRN, OvaCheck).

In our opinion, single identified biomarkers or panels of these are more useful in contrast to pattern recognition, because

- differences in peptide expression levels can be assigned in multiple biological sources such as tumour tissue, blood, urine;
- the test validation can be performed on another detection system (e.g. immunoassays);
- a biological hypothesis can be generated and validated;
- established and approved clinical validation procedures can be used.

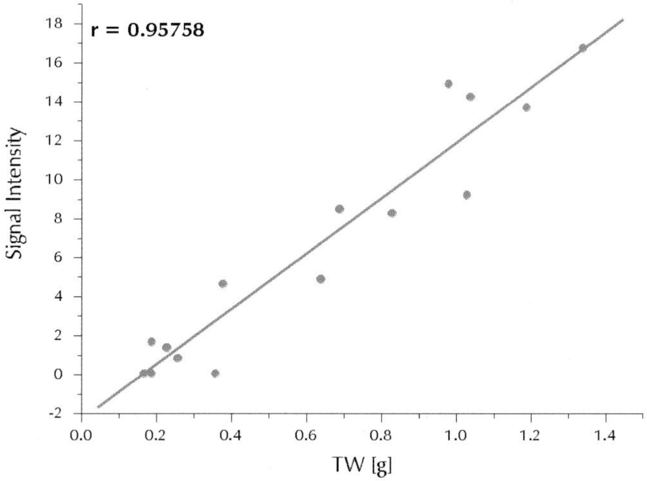

Fig. 40: Correlation between tumour weight and MALDI MS signal intensity.
The graph depicts the correlation between the tumour weight and the corresponding signal intensity of human TIF-1ß.

A marker released from tumour tissue will undergo a significant dilution process on its way into the blood stream. The likelihood for tumour marker discovery depends on a combination of the concentration of the marker, and the sensitivity of the detection method in a complex biological sample. The direct analysis and comparison of plasma samples from controls and cancer patients requires sensitivity down to the low pM range. Nowadays multiplex systems based on mass spectrometry do not permit such sensitive detection of endogenous plasma peptides. As a result, at the moment a discovery strategy should integrate the analysis of model systems, tumour and control tissue as well as body fluids to enhance sensitivity (Fig. 38-40). The challenge over the next years is to promote such integrative approaches and improve the sensitivity of multiplex systems.

2.6 Characterisation of the Urinary Peptidome

Michael Jürgens, Annette Appel, Susanne Neitz, Gabriele Heine, and Christoph Menzel

2.6.1 Introduction

Urinalysis has a long history in medicinal diagnostics reaching back at least 2000 years to ancient Egypt, where polyuria and haematuria are mentioned as stages of disease in old medical papyri. Today, urine test stripes are a central diagnostic instrument with a major importance in first-line diagnostics. Typically, early symptoms of three groups are detected: (i) diseases of the kidneys and the urinary tract, (ii) carbohydrate metabolism disorders (diabetes mellitus), and (iii) liver diseases and haemolytic disorders [59].

2.6.2 Biomarker research in urine

With the advent of the general discussion about the necessity of new biomarkers, also biomarker discovery in human urine has become an evolving and potentially valuable field of study especially in relation to renal function and diseases of the urinary tract [60]. In order to deliver on the promises and to facilitate the development of validated biomarkers or biomarker panels, protein profiling techniques need high sample throughput, speed of analysis, and reproducibility of results. Here we outline the performance characteristics of peptidomics technologies, namely the liquid chromatography/MALDI-TOF-MS based differential peptide display (DPD) approach for separating, detecting, abundance profiling and identification of native peptides [1] derived from human urine. The typical complexity of human urine (resolution of the technique with respect to the detectable number of peptides), the reproducibility of the technique (coefficient of variation for abundance profiles of all peptides detected in biological samples), the dynamic range of the technique as well as the limit of detection were characterised for the specimen urine.

2.6.3 Methods

For clinical chemical analysis, different urine specimens are used (spontaneous, first morning, timed urine etc.) depending on test purpose. We decided to use the midstream portion of first morning urine as it should ensure sufficiently long residence in the bladder, a composition independent of daily variations due to food and fluid intake, and physical activity. In addition, sample volumes used for analysis are normalised to urinary creatinine concentrations as most peptides' and proteins' reference values are given with respect to urinary creatinine (e.g. albumin, alpha-amylase, IgG, alpha-1-acid glycoprotein, transferrin). After normalisation, peptides and small proteins with a molecular mass of up to approximately 15 kDa were extracted from urine of female and

	Mean coefficient of variation (%)	Mean coefficient of variation (%) of mean signal intensity of a peptide map
a) Pooled urine	39.4	5.2
b) Individual urine samples	62.3	9.1

Table 3: General descriptive statistics for performance characteristics of DPD.
Applied to a) pooled human urinary samples: 10 individual samples from female and male healthy donors each were pooled prior to analysis; subsequently 20 aliquots of the urine pool were subjected to peptide chemical and biostatistic analysis; b) statistics for individual human urinary samples: 10 individual samples from female and male healthy donors each were subjected in duplicates to peptide chemical and biostatistic analysis.

male healthy volunteers. In addition, urine samples from patients suffering from post-renal filtering diseases (nephrolithiasis, prostate and bladder cancer) were used after having obtained the patients' written informed consent. Samples were separated by HPLC and collected fractions were analysed individually by MALDI-TOF-MS. Spectrometric data were transferred to a database to compose peptide profiles of individual samples and to calculate peptide master displays representing the peptidome of defined groups of samples. A substantial number of peptides present in a master display was identified as landmarks for normal human urine applying direct "top-down" mass spectrometric sequencing by state-of-the-art analytical instrumentation as described in detail elsewhere [28]. In addition, classical N-terminal Edman sequencing has been used after purification of some larger peptides and for peptides not amenable to mass spectrometric sequencing.

2.6.4 Results

Using pooled urine of 10 male and female healthy volunteers each, a peptide master display was created resolving about 7,000 signal coordinates. These signal coordinates are extracted to constitute the general position list used for further analysis. Replicate measurements of the respective urine pool displayed an average coefficient of variation (CV) for each signal coordinate of 39.4%, whereas the mean signal intensity for all coordinates within an individual map had a CV of 5.2%. Using individual urine samples measured in duplicates, the CV values rose to 62.3 % (average for each coordinate) and 9.1 % (mean intensity of maps) respectively (cf. Table 3). These performance characteristics can now be used for power calculations in biomarker discovery projects. After spiking of the urine pool with a mixture of 13 peptides in concentrations from 440 pmol/L to 7 nmol/L (theoretical in vivo concentrations with respect to the applied urinary

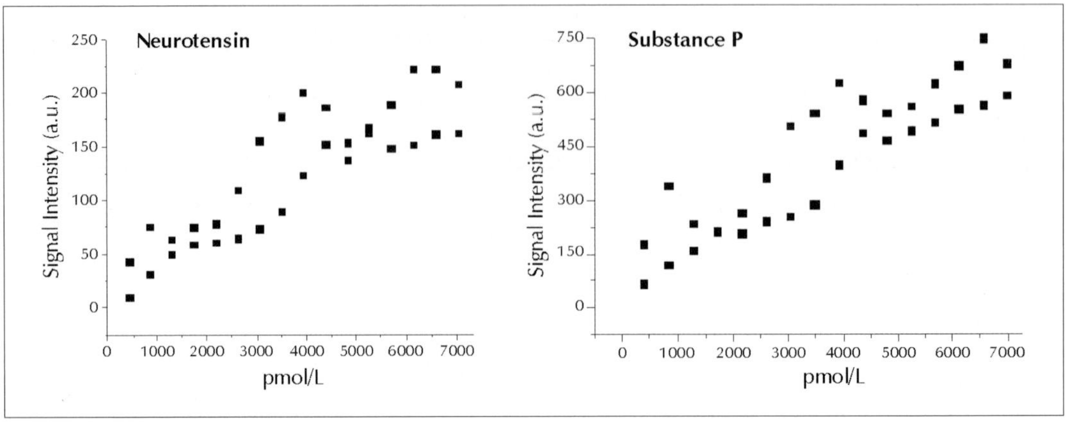

Fig. 41: Quantification capability of DPD abundance profiling within urine.
Aliquots from a pool of normal urine were spiked with 13 standard peptides in concentrations from 440 pmol/L to 7.04 nmol/L (theoretical in vivo concentrations with respect to the applied urinary volume used for analysis) and measured in duplicates. The signal readouts for Neurotensin (left panel) and Substance P (right panel) are displayed exemplarily. Note that, though signal intensities differ approximately 3-fold between the peptides, both peptides are a) detectable at the lowest concentration applied and moreover b) the dynamic range for (semi-) quantitative analysis is comparable.

volume used for analysis) correlation analysis of signal intensities to concentration of spiked peptides revealed that only the signals of the standard peptides reached r-values > 0.8. This result clearly demonstrates the quantification capability of the approach. The limit of detection (LOD) and the dynamic range are generally depending on the individual peptide/signal coordinate: LOD for typical peptides such as Substance P or Neurotensin is at or below 500 pmol/L with a dynamic range of detection of between 1 to 3 orders of magnitude (Fig. 41).

More than 150 individual peptides derived from about 70 protein precursors have been identified in normal urine (Fig. 42). Though many precursors are known as blood plasma derived, the subcellular location of a substantial number is extracellular, vesicular/lysosomal, intracellular or within the cell membrane. Comparing these identifications to different urine proteome studies [61-63], the results are in good agreement. In addition to reflecting those proteins which are addressable by typical proteomic techniques, peptidomics also shows the turnover of very large proteins, e.g. collagens, by their degradation products. Moreover, small proteins and peptides like the class of defensins can be shown in their processed form almost exclusively applying peptidomics methods as they are cleaved from their larger protein precursors. In addition, post-translational modifications like oxidations of proline and lysine residues in e.g. collagens, glycosylation in e.g. alpha-2-HS-glycoprotein or phosphorylation in e.g. Osteopontin can be shown and often be matched to the exact site of modification.

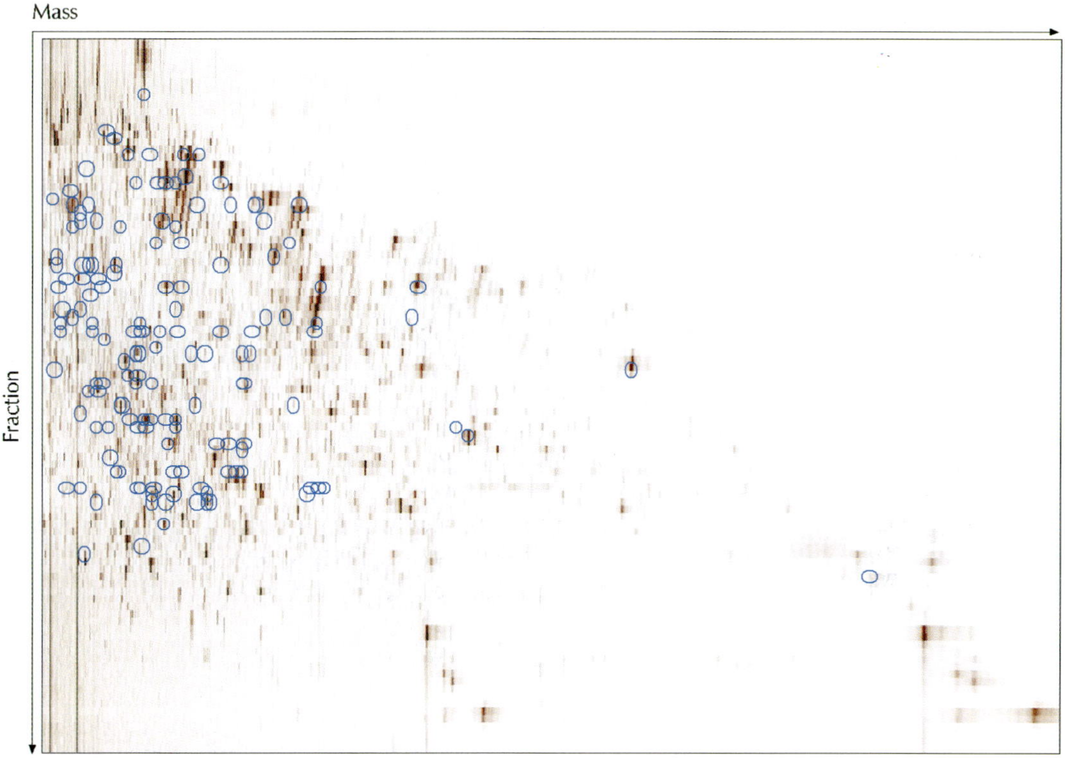

Fig. 42: Annotated peptide map from urine.
Mapping of over 150 different peptides from about 70 protein precursors sequenced from normal human urine so far. The approach attempts to know a basic set of peptides, which as "landmarks" qualify to describe the peptidic content of normal human urine. These sets of peptides can then be used to assist sequencing of signal coordinates of interest within biomarker discovery studies, e.g. in comparison with pathologic urine.

For illustration purposes, we have screened urines from patients suffering from post-renal filtration diseases. Many features known from normal urines are also present in these pathological samples meaning that their general peptide pattern can easily be attributed to the specimen urine. However, huge qualitative differences are obvious even by visual comparison of the respective mean peptide displays (Fig. 43; see page 82).

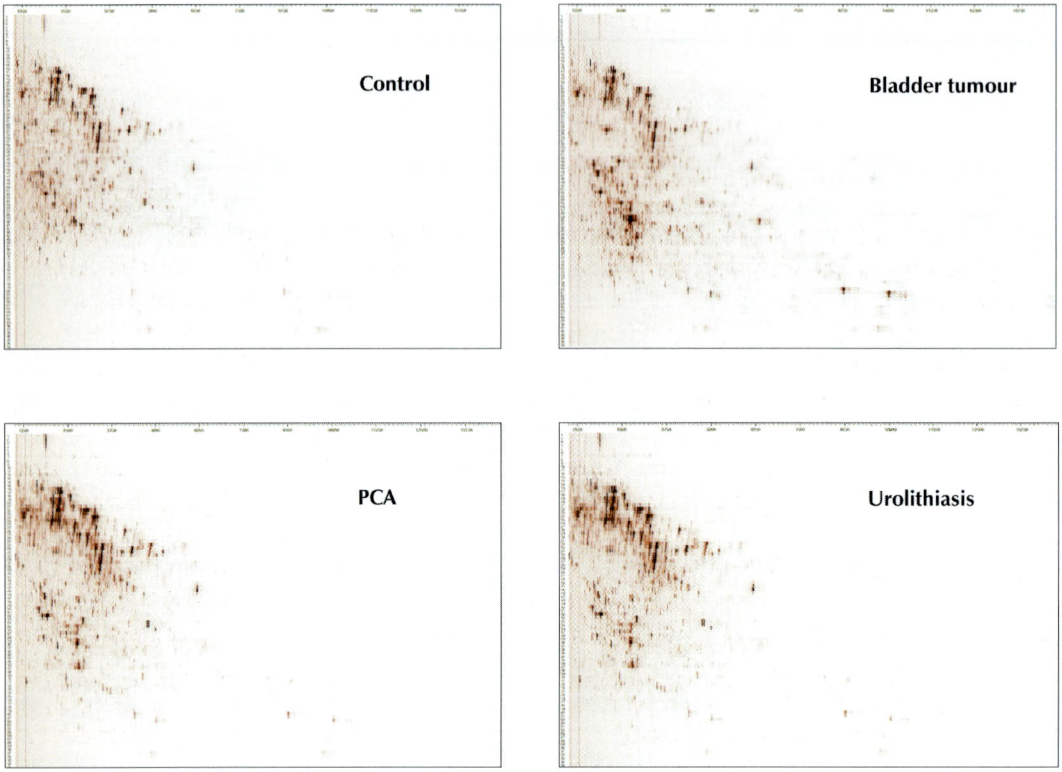

Fig. 43: Urine pathologies.

Global view on mean maps of normal urine, urine from bladder tumour patients, urine from patients with a diagnosis of urolithiasis and urine from patients suffering from prostate cancer (clockwise from top left). Though some general features of urine are consistent with the peptide displays, qualitative differences between the different pathologic states are easily revealed.

2.6.5 Conclusion

The peptidomics technology has a great potential for high-throughput, high-resolution urine peptide profiling analyses as shown in this investigation. It is not only a promising tool to study renal physiology and pathophysiology and to determine new biomarkers of renal diseases, but it also has the potential to study remotely localised or systemic aberrations within human biology.

2.7 Peptidomics and Diabetes

Petra Budde,
Imke Schulte,
Hartmut Selle,
and Horst Rose

Over the past 25 years the prevalence of type 2 diabetes has increased dramatically throughout the world [64]. The main driving forces are obesity due to unhealthy lifestyles, with overeating as a dominant feature, and population aging. Worldwide changes in lifestyle accelerate the incidence of diabetes also in developing nations: In 2025 the projected number of diabetics will be largest in India (> 57 million), followed by China (> 37 million) and can thus be expected to outnumber the United States (> 21 million). Type 2 diabetes is a life threatening disease which is associated with an increased incidence of stroke, heart failure, blindness, limb amputations and end-stage renal disease (ESRD). In a simplified way type 2 diabetes can be explained as a combination of (i) insulin resistance defined as the reduced ability of insulin to stimulate glucose uptake and to suppress hepatic glucose output and (ii) defects in insulin secretion. In a prediabetic state the pancreatic beta-cells compensate for the relative insulin deficiency by insulin hypersecretion, but eventually fail to match the degree of insulin resistance (hypoinsulinaemia). Diabetes often remains undiagnosed until the progress of the disease leads to obvious late-stage diabetic complications. Thus, early detection and adequate therapy to improve insulin sensitivity are important to prevent the development of new-onset diabetes and late-stage complications.

The precursor disease of type 2 diabetes is the so-called *metabolic syndrome* or *syndrome X* [65]. The World Health Organization (WHO) was the first to publish an internationally accepted definition for metabolic syndrome in 1998, but the criteria that have received the most widespread acceptance and use are those proposed as part of ATP III (the third report of the National Cholesterol Education Program expert panel on Detection, Evaluation, and Treatment of High Blood Cholesterol in Adults). ATP III defines the metabolic syndrome as involving three or more of the following components that provide useful criteria to identify individuals at increased risk to develop type 2 diabetes and cardiovascular disease [66]:

- Central obesity (waist circumference >102 cm in men, > 88 cm in women)
- Fasting triglycerides (≥150 mg/dL)
- HDL cholesterol (<40 mg/dL in men, <50 mg/dL in women)
- Blood pressure (≥130/85 mm Hg)
- Fasting glucose (≥10 mg/dL)

All of the factors associated with metabolic syndrome are interrelated. However, because of the dramatic and parallel increase of diabetes and obesity, the latter is often regarded as being mainly responsible for the rising prevalence of the metabolic syndrome. Obesity and lack of exercise enhance insulin resistance and metabolic syndrome. In the US, it is estimated that 20% of adults (about 47 million) have metabolic syndrome. About 5.4

million persons (2.7%) have fasting plasma glucose ≥ 126 mg/dL, and 13.4 million (6.9%) have impaired fasting glucose (110 to 125 mg/dL). Alongside with a rising occurrence of the metabolic syndrome, a rising frequency in gestational diabetes is observed. As the main causes, an altered glucose metabolism together with decreased insulin sensitivity and obesity are named. Although the underlying mechanisms still need to be elucidated, the risk for developing obesity and type 2 diabetes later in life is increased for the child as well as for the mother [67].

The WHO recommends to detect abnormal glucose tolerance by an Oral Glucose Tolerance Test (OGTT) using a 75-g glucose load. Abnormal glucose tolerance detected by an OGTT, despite its limitations, conveys important prognostic information not disclosed by other risk factors or measurements. The use of an OGTT to identify patients at risk to develop cardiovascular disease and diabetes is under debate. The main concern is the inconvenience and relative high cost of OGTT in clinical practice. Efforts to screen for more reliable biomarkers that would substitute the OGTT are important to improve the assessment of cardiovascular and diabetes risks of overweight and obese patients.

2.7.1 Peptides and the metabolic syndrome

What mechanisms are involved by which obesity causes insulin resistance and what are the key factors leading to type 2 diabetes and cardiovascular disease?

Two separate mechanisms have been proposed that may have some degree of interrelation:

(i) The sustained imbalance between caloric intake and energy consumption causes excess fat (adipose) tissue that has a higher rate of lipolysis. The products of lipolysis, free fatty acids (FFA), are believed to cause muscle insulin resistance and decrease the ability of insulin to suppress lipolysis.

(ii) Besides energy storage adipose tissue is an active endocrine organ that secretes a great number of several newly discovered hormones, called adipokines, including leptin, resistin, adipsin and adiponectin [68]. These adipokines are actively involved in regulating insulin sensitivity, energy homoeostasis and food consumption (Please refer to chapter 2.9.2 for more information). With increasing adipose tissue size and mass the secretory profile and cellular homeostasis become dysregulated. Qualitative and quantitative changes in the expression of proinflammatory cytokines contribute to systemic insulin resistance and cardiovascular diseases. In summary, hormonal factors secreted by adipose tissue exacerbate insulin resistance ultimately leading to type 2 diabetes. However, the question of how beta-cells fail to compensate long-term insulin resistance remains largely unanswered.

The detection of early abnormalities of beta-cell function is crucial to prevent the progression from impaired glucose tolerance to type 2 diabetes. However, the earliest insulin secretory defects in the progression from normal to abnormal glucose tolerance may be subtle. Insulin is the principal hormone responsible for the control of glucose metabolism. It is synthesised in the beta-cells of the islets of Langerhans as the precursor, proinsulin, which is processed to form C-peptide and insulin. As diagnostic tool the secretory functions of the pancreatic beta cells are tested by determining proinsulin, insulin and C-peptide concentrations. A disproportion in the relative concentrations of circulating proinsulin (and proinsulin intermediates) to insulin was shown to be a feature of later stages of type 2 diabetes [69]. It has been speculated that the increased demand on insulin due to obesity and/or insulin resistance may result in secretion of immature beta-cell granules with a higher content of proinsulin. Another peptide hormone of the beta-cell, amylin (islet amyloid polypeptide, IAPP) has also been implicated in the progressive beta cell failure in type 2 diabetes mellitus. Amylin has been shown to be the precursor for the amyloid deposits frequently observed in patients with type 2 diabetes.

Peptide hormones or incretins released from the gut also play an important role in augmenting the glucose stimulated insulin secretion. Because this effect occurs after meal ingestion it has been termed as the incretin response. The major peptide hormones responsible for the incretin effect are glucose dependent insulinotropic polypeptide (GIP) and glucagon-like peptide-1 (GLP-1). GLP-1 has great potential in the treatment of type 2 diabetes because it stimulates insulin secretion and biosynthesis, inhibits glucagon secretion, hepatic glucose production and reduces beta-cell apoptosis (Table 4; see page 87). Experiments in diabetic patients and those with impaired glucose tolerance have shown a dysregulated incretin response which may also contribute to the pathophysiology of type 2 diabetes. In summary, despite upcoming peptide biomarkers that indicate a disturbed incretin response and significant deterioration of beta-cell secretion, early biomarkers that provide the clinical diagnosis of insulin resistance and secretion disorder suitable in general practice are missing.

2.7.2 Peptides as drugs in pharmaceutical applications

A number of new approaches to treat diabetes are currently undergoing clinical trials, including those involving stimulation of the pancreatic beta-cell with bioactive peptides such as GLP-1 and amylin. GLP-1 based therapies are attractive because GLP-1 action on insulin secretion is strictly glucose dependent and hypoglycaemia does not develop during GLP-1 application (Table 4; see page 87). However, to be clinically useful, GLP-1 has to be protected from rapid degradation by dipeptidyl peptidase IV (DPPIV), the major enzyme responsible for degrading the incretins *in vivo* [70]. An opposite approach is to delay incretin degradation by inhibiting DPPIV. Several DPPIV inhibitors are currently being explored as a new approach to increase the physiological actions of incretin hormones in the treatment of type 2 diabetes [71]. In addition to their therapeutic effects, chronic treatment with DPPIV inhibitors requires comprehensive knowledge regarding the selectivity of the inhibitors. Section 2.4 outlines in detail how DPPIV peptide substrates can be identified from plasma samples in vivo.

The discovery of new bioactive peptides is a subject of extensive research and development programmes in the field of diabetes and obesity. In obesity therapy one major focus is on the regulation of peptides and the corresponding receptors involved in central appetite regulation. To increase insulin sensitivity is another strategy addressed by researchers in academia and pharmaceutical companies evaluating peptides like adiponectin that control peripheral insulin sensitivity and fat metabolism. As in other chronic diseases, long-term use of prescription medications is often limited by side effects. Clearly, novel therapeutic tools that are well-tolerated but achieve improved glycaemic control without increasing the risk of hypoglycemia and weight gain are urgently needed. Peptides offer intrinsic advantages in this respect. They are naturally found in the human body and, if administered properly, are supposed to have fewer adverse side effects in their native form than small molecule compounds. By using the native form of a peptide, which generally bears only a low risk of adverse immunologic reaction, the development time to advance a drug candidate into clinical trials can be reduced.

In a survey in relevant databases a range of products currently under development for diabetes therapy are found; examples are given in Table 4.

2.7.3 Peptidomics for biomarkers and drug discovery

Peptide hormones, like insulin and glucagon play a key role in the pathophysiology and diagnosis of diabetes type 2. Peptidomics, especially the technology of *Differential Peptide Display* (DPD) matches the molecular mass window of peptide hormones and biomarkers. A proof-of-principle study was conducted to demonstrate that DPD is an attractive approach to develop biomarkers for the early diagnosis of impaired glucose tolerance that may eventually replace the laborious OGTT.

Sensitive detection of peptide hormones

A study was conducted with healthy subjects to detect plasma peptides responding to an oral glucose provocation test. Applying DPD we detected ~20 peptides that changed in response to an oral glucose challenge (Fig. 44; see page 88). Among the identified peptides whose relative abundance increased significantly were peptide hormones that are important to maintain glucose homoestasis such as insulin and its corresponding C-peptide. Measurements of circulating levels of insulin and C-peptide by ELISA before and after glucose challenge confirmed that the increase of candidate peptides determinded by mass spectrometry reflects the actual increase in plasma (Fig. 45; see page 89). We can thus demonstrate that peptidomics technologies can match the sensitivity required to determine altered levels of peptide hormones in the picomolar range.

Development phase	Compound	Indication	Company
Discovery	Ghrelin	Type 2 diabetes	Theratechnologies
	EN122001, Insulin enhancing novel peptide hormone	Type 2 diabetes	Protemix
Preclinical	EN122004, Peptide hormone for suppression of insulin resistance	Type 2 diabetes	Protemix
	ThGLP-1, GLP-1 analogue	Type 2 diabetes	Theratechnologies
	Peptide YY 3-36	Obesity	Amylin
	PTP-1B Inhibitor	Diabetes/obesity	Serono
Phase I	GLP1-I.N.T., combination of GLP-1 and gastrin analogue (G1)	IDDM	Transition Therapeutics
Phase I/II a	ZP10, GLP-1 analogue	Type 2 diabetes	Zealand/Aventis
Phase II	DiaPep227	Autoimmune diabetes	Develogen
	ThGRF	Type 2 diabetes	Theratechnologies
	BIM 51077	Type 2 diabetes	Ipsen
Phase II	Exenatide LAR Liraglutide, GLP-1 derivative	Type 2 diabetes	Novo Nordisk
Phase III	Synthetic exendin-4, incretin-mimetic agent	Type 1 and 2 diabetes	Amylin/Lilly
Approval	Symlin, synthetic version of the human hormone amylin	Type 2 diabetes	Amylin
Exenatide LAR	Axokine, modified form of naturally occurring protein, Ciliary Neurotrophic Factor	Obesity	Regeneron

Table 4: Examples for new diabetes or obesity drugs currently under development.

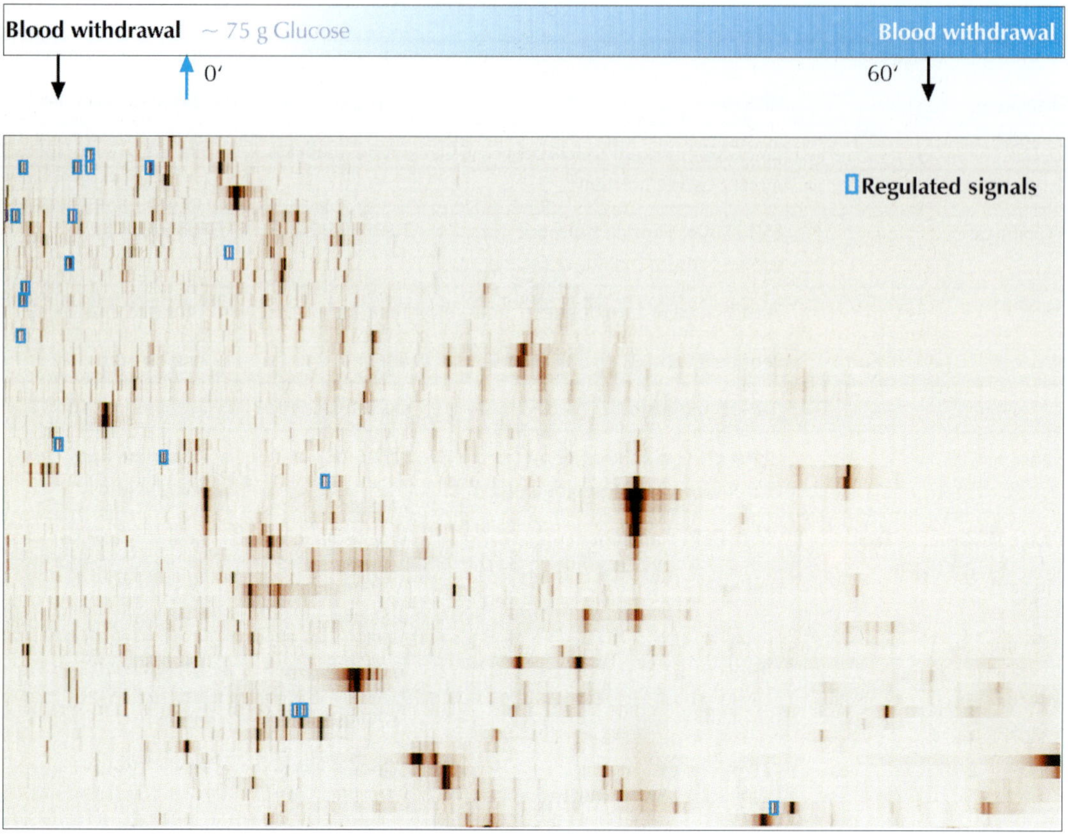

Fig. 44: Changes in endogenous peptides after oral glucose challenge.
Endogenous peptides were stimulated in healthy individuals by oral glucose challenge (upper sketch). Changes in endogenous peptide concentrations (blue squares) were followed in order to validate the concept by detecting meaningful biomarkers that are clearly related to the challenge.

In combination with a specific drug challenge, a broad set of applications in preclinical and clinical settings seem feasible. This would open up enormous potential in the course of drug development to bridge findings from animal models into early phase clinical trials.

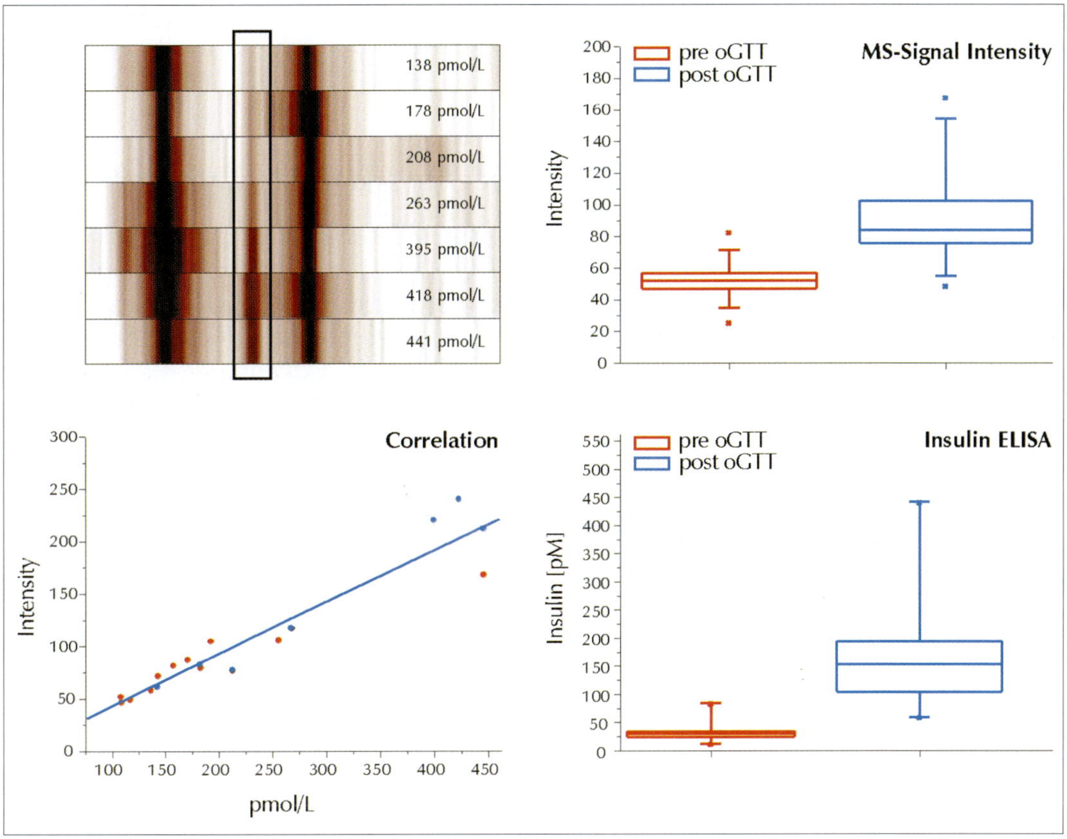

Fig. 45: Changes in insulin and C-peptide after oral glucose challenge.

Left: Selected mass spectra which represent different concentrations of plasma insulin (boxed) are shown. The actual plasma concentration of insulin is depicted on the left side.

Correlation of MS signal intensities of insulin versus plasma concentrations determined by ELISA. The r-value is > 0.9.

Right: Box- and Whisker plots of mass spectrometric signals of insulin (upper panel) and their plasma levels determined by ELISA (lower panel) before and after oral glucose challenge.

2.8 Mouse Models of Obesity and Type 2 Diabetes

Petra Budde

2.8.1 Classic mouse and rat models in obesity and diabetes research

Laboratory animals are extensively used in academic institutions and the pharmaceutical industry as exploratory models to understand the basic mechanisms leading to the development of type 2 diabetes and its associated complications [72, 73]. However, being complex metabolic diseases, obesity and type 2 diabetes pose a difficult challenge to identify the most promising targets for drug development. Explanatory mouse models could help to unravel the contribution of environmental and genetic factors to the disease progression.

Before the development of transgenic and knock-out mouse technology, the majority of obesity and diabetes mouse models were naturally occurring genetic mutations in inbred strains [74]. The most famous example is the obese *(ob/ob)* mouse observed in 1949 at the Jackson Laboratory (http://www.jax.org). Interest in the research area exploded when the obesity mutation was mapped to the adipose tissue hormone leptin (14 kDa) [75, 76] that acts as an appetite suppressant in the brain. Another spontaneous mouse mutant, the diabetic *(db/db)* mouse was discovered in 1966 at the Jackson Laboratories and lacks functional leptin receptors. When recombinant leptin was injected in *ob/ob* mice they immediately lost weight [77]. Unlike in mice overweight humans have increased leptin levels and appear to be resistant to the hormone. Although disappointing, the leptin story contributed enormously to the understanding how and which hormonal circuits in the brain control energy homoeostasis, feeding behaviour and body weight. A summary of the classical rodent obesity and type 2 diabetes models is presented in Table 5.

2.8.2 Differential peptidomics of obesity and diabetes mouse models

For decades these mice were extremely instructive for studying the effects of obesity and overeating on insulin production and action in liver, muscle and adipose tissue. Gene expression studies in insulin sensitive tissues have clearly helped to identify novel targets that modulate insulin action. Less frequently emphasised is that type 2 diabetes and obesity also affect the level of peptide hormones in endocrine tissues such as gut [71], pancreas, hypothalamus [78] and adipose tissue [68].

In a first attempt, we analysed peptides from all tissues in mice that are relevant for the development of obesity and diabetes (Fig. 46).

Considering that the major pancreatic hormones, insulin, glucagon and islet amyloid polypeptide (IAPP, amylin) are peptides released from larger precursors, peptidomics represents a direct and elegant technology to identify diabetes related alterations in the peptide composition of the pancreas. Under conditions of enhanced stress, such as elevated blood glucose and lipid levels, the pancreatic beta-cells from obese mice respond with a compensatory upregulation of the insulin biosynthesis rate (proinsulin, Fig. 47; see page 92).

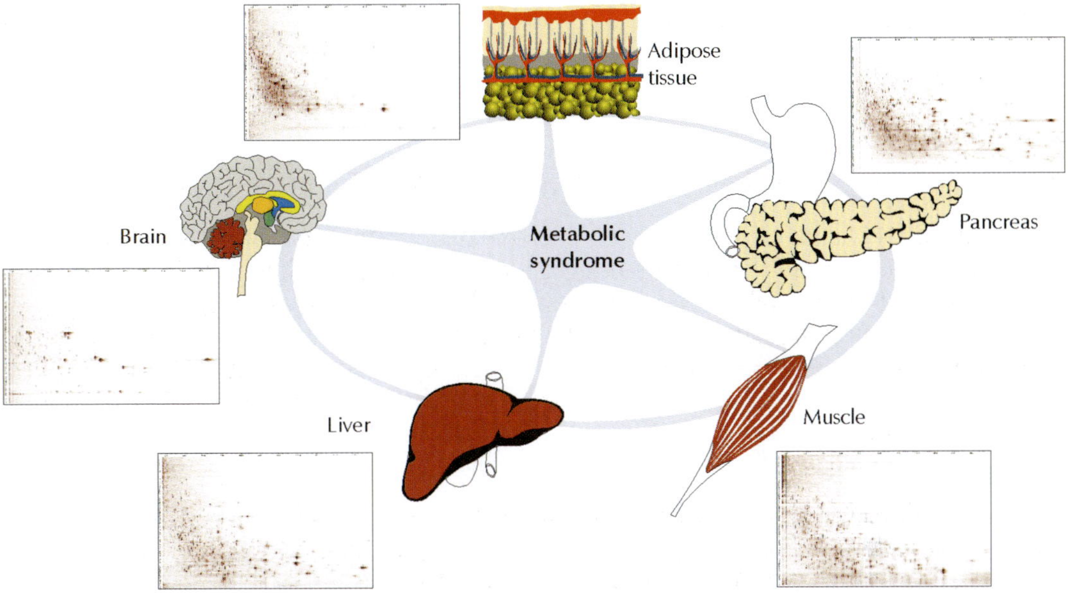

Fig. 46: Multi-organ involvement in metabolic syndrome.
Peptide displays of peptidomes from brain, skeletal muscle, liver, adipose tissue and pancreas from mouse. From sample amounts from 1 – 10 mg more than 5,000 endogenous peptides are displayed. All tissues have distinctly different peptide composition.

Mutation	Primary Defect	Phenotype	Application
Obese (lep^{ob}/lep^{ob} mouse)	Nonsense mutation in the adipose tissue derived hormone leptin prevents its inhibitory effect on food intake	Obesity, hyperphagia, transient hyperglycaemia, hyperinsulinaemia, insulin resistance	Preclinical model for obesity and insulin resistance
Diabetes ($lepr^{db}/lepr^{db}$ mouse)	Mutation in the leptin receptor gene causes defective leptin signalling	The clinical symptoms and course of the disease are more severe than in the ob/ob mouse	Preclinical model for type 2 diabetes
Fatty (Zucker fa/fa rat)	Leptin receptor	Obesity, insulin resistance, hyperinsulinaemia	Preclinical model for obesity and insulin resistance
Fat (cpe^{fat}/cpe^{fat} mouse)	A mutation in the carboxypeptidase E gene causes defective prohormone processing	Obesity, hyperglycaemia, insulin resistance, hyperinsulinaemia	Discovery of neuroendocrine peptides involved in the pathogenesis of obesity and insulin resistance

Table 5: Rodent obesity and type 2 diabetes models.

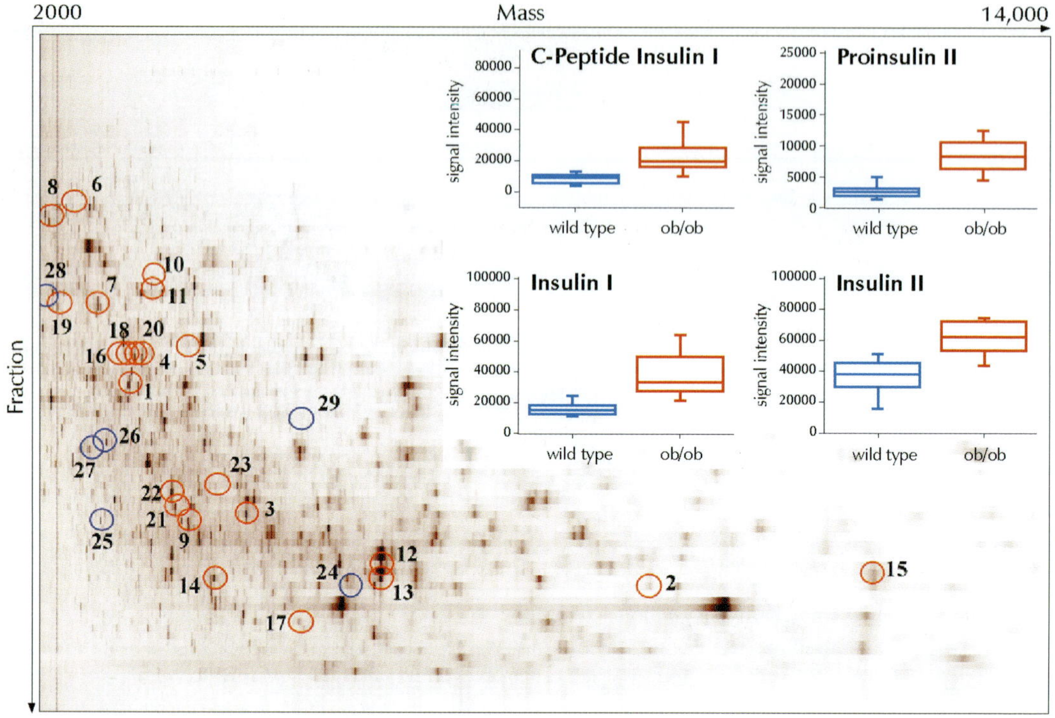

Fig. 47: Peptidomics profiling of pancreas from ob/ob mice.
The peptide master display of pancreas with identified peptide hormones that increased in obese mice. A differential peptidomics analysis of pancreas from control and obese *(ob/ob)* mice was carried out to study changes in the levels of peptides as a result of obesity and insulin resistance. Compared to control mice, obese mice exhibit increased production of proinsulin and other peptide hormones causing a hyperinsulinaemic phenotype.

The net result would be an increase in the insulin secretory capacity of the beta-cell that can be visualised and quantified by peptidomics. In addition to insulin, obesity also affects the production of other polypeptides, such as the 37 amino acid peptide hormone amylin (islet amyloid polypeptide, IAPP). Amylin is co-stored with insulin in secretory granules of pancreatic islet beta-cells and is the primary constituent of the islet amyloid that develops in human type 2 diabetes. Thus, the peptidomic approach has the potential to unravel novel biomarkers of early pancreatic stress. The normalisation of these changes can be further utilised in testing how antidiabetic drugs improve beta-cell function.

An opposite approach to the analysis of secondary effects of obesity (or more precisely impaired leptin signalling) on peptide hormones is to study how defects in peptide hormone biosynthesis affect body weight and glucose metabolism. In the mid 90's another gene on chromosome 8 in mice that affects obesity and diabetes was discovered at the Jackson Laboratories, a Ben Harbor, ME (USA) based mammalian genetic research facility. Mice bearing the so-called "fat" mutation are obese and have elevated blood glucose levels, but treatment of these mice with insulin normalised blood glucose levels [79, 80].

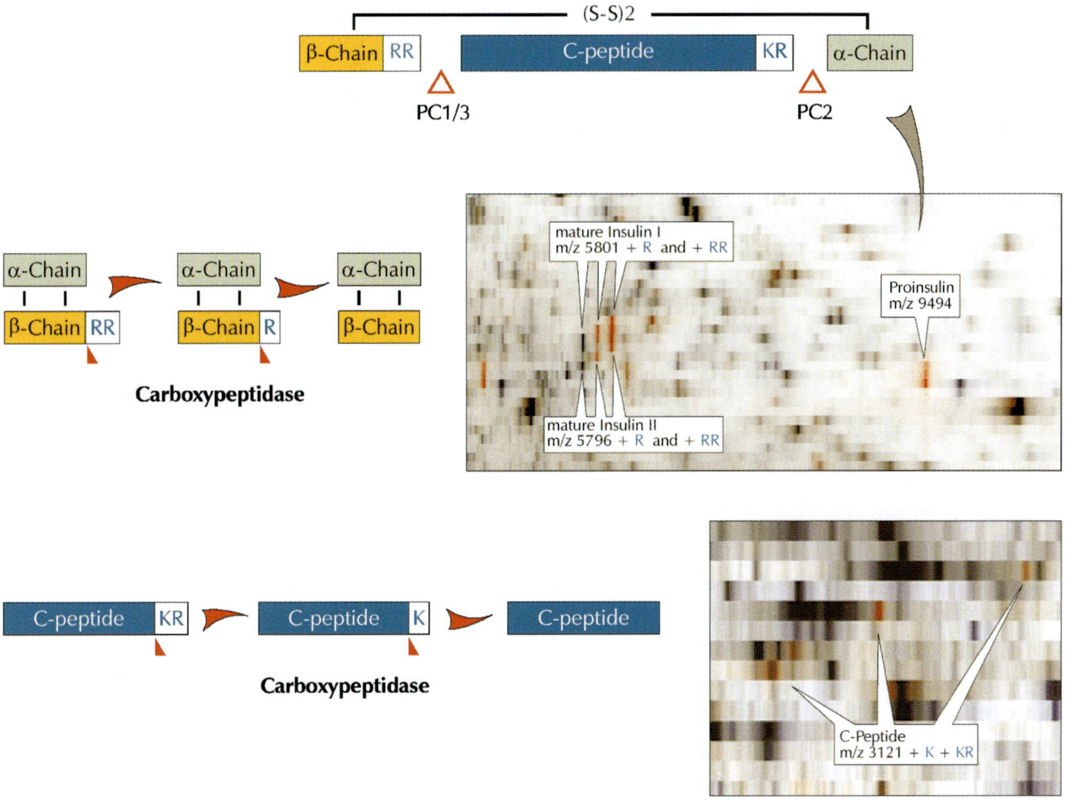

Fig. 48: Impaired prohormone processing in fat/fat mice.
Identification of incompletely processed peptide hormones from *fat/fat* mice using peptidomics. *Fat/fat* mice are obese and have elevated plasma glucose levels and carry a mutation in the carboxypeptidase E gene, a peptidase located in the processing pathway of peptide hormones. As a consequence, these mice exhibit a characteristic pattern of peptide hormone intermediates having additional basic amino acids at their carboxy terminus. This is exemplified for the processing pathway of proinsulin. As a consequence of the mutation, *fat/fat* mice accumulate and secrete less active proinsulin, causing a phenotype of hyperproinsulinaemia.

Apparently, the *fat/fat* mice are not insulin resistant and a residual insulin secretion is preserved. What might be the underlying molecular defect? It became evident, as seen from figure 48, that these mice exhibit a significant disproportion between the less active insulin precursor and the downstream product of several processing steps, mature insulin. What emerged was a fascinating molecular defect in the prohormone processing pathway in *fat/fat* mice. Subsequently, the mutation was mapped to carboxypeptidase E (CPE), an enzyme that trims off basic amino acids remaining after cleavage of prohormone processing enzymes [80]. Those findings called enormous attraction to study the processing pathway of peptide hormones using different approaches [81–84]. We conducted an in-depth peptidomics study of pancreatic tissue and found impaired albeit not absent carboxypeptidase activity. As seen in the experiments of Fig. 48 the point mutation in CPE resulted in increased levels of insulin as well as glucagon and amylin processing intermediates with additional basic amino acids at their carboxy terminus. This, however, did not cause the complete deficiency of mature peptide hormones. The mechanisms through which the endocrine pancreas accomplishes a minimum level of active peptide hormones before developing diabetes still remain elusive. A likely explanation might be a compensatory upregulation of another carboxypeptidase. As a polygenic disorder, equivalent monogenetic defects related to obesity are rare in humans. However, the *fat/fat* mice have opened insight in the biosynthesis pathway of key peptides regulating metabolism and body weight.

2.8.3 Obesity and diabetes mouse models in preclinical studies

Finally, another important usage of the classical diabetes rodent models is the *in vivo* testing of novel antidiabetic drugs (Table 6). To predict a beneficial therapeutic effect or to assess toxicity it is of importance that the mouse model closely resembles the pathology of the human disease. It might be argued that the fidelity between monogenic mouse models and the polygenic nature of human type 2 diabetes is only poor. However, regarding the physiological outcome of diabetic drug intervention both *ob/ob* and *db/db* have proven to be useful preclinical mouse models. At present, novel and upcoming antidiabetic drugs rely mainly on the following approaches: (i) enhancement of insulin action (peroxisome proliferator activated receptor-, PPARγ agonists, thiazolidinediones) or (ii) enhancement of glucose stimulated insulin secretion. The latter approach aims to improve the action of the intestinal glucagon-like peptide 1 (GLP-1) and glucose dependent insulinotropic peptide (GIP), responsible for stimulation insulin secretion by beta-cells in response to food [70]. The half-life and bioactivity of these peptides is tightly regulated by peptidase IV (DPPIV) that specifically cleaves off X-Pro or X-Ala from the amino terminus. DPPIV-resistant GLP-1 analogues reduced the glycaemic levels in a number of preclinical models (*ob/ob* and *db/db* mice) and increased beta-cell mass and proliferation [85-88]. An opposite rational strategy is to increase the action of endogenous GLP-1 by inhibiting DPPIV (reviewed in [70]). DPPIV inhibitors potentiate the action of GLP-1 and GIP in *db/db* mice [89] or obese Zucker (*fa/fa*) rats [90] and moderately improve insulin resistance. Several major pharmaceutical companies (Novartis, Merck, GlaxoSmithKline, Prosidion, Bristol-Myers Squibb) have developed DPPIV inhibitors that are currently in clinical development [91]. DPPIV was originally discovered as a T-lymphocyte surface glycoprotein, designated CD26, but is widely distributed in numerous tissues. DPPIV has diverse functional properties, such as immune regulation, signal transduction, apoptosis and tumour progression (reviewed in [92]). The substrates are growth factors, chemokines, neuropeptides, and vasoactive peptides. Targeting the proteolytic activity of DPPIV has many promising therapeutic potentials and may prompt the development of highly selective inhibitors. A peptidomics study has been conducted to test the specificity of DPPIV inhibitors in preclinical animal models (for detailed information please refer to chapter 2.4.7). This will add data on target functions and define pathways affected by inhibitors, providing a useful approach to assess the risk of side effects. This study may help to reduce attrition in costly clinical trials.

Target	Knock-out models	Validation in diabetic rodents	Mechanisms	Therapeutic application	Developmental stage
DPPIV (CD26): Aminopeptidase involved in the breakdown of peptide hormones and cytokines	Increased incretin hormone levels in $CD26^{-/-}$ and $GLP\text{-}1^{-/-}$ mice	*db/db* mice Zucker *fa/fa* rats	DPPIV inhibitors prolong the action of blood glucose lowering incretin hormones. Effects on further DPPIV substrates expected	Type 2 diabetes hyperglycaemia	Clincial studies
GLP-1 analogues: Intestinal peptide hormone stimulates insulin secretion and β-cell survival	Fasting hyperglycaemia in GLP-1 receptor k.o. mice, abnormal oral glucose tolerance	*ob/ob* mice *db/db* mice Zucker *fa/fa* rats	Prolonged clucose lowering activity by improved stability of GLP-1 analogues	Type 2 diabetes hyperglycaemia	Clincial studies
PPARγ agonists: Nuclear receptor controls adipose differentiation, expression of adipokines, glucose and lipid metabolism	Improved insulin sensitivity, resistance to obesity in $PPAR\gamma^{+/-}$ mice	*ob/ob* mice *db/db* mice Zucker *fa/fa* rats	PPARγ agonists (thiazolidinedione) improve insulin sensitivity, glucose lowering and anti-inflammatory action	Insulin resistance Type 2 diabetes	At market, second generation in preclinical and clinical studies

Table 6: Diabetes rodent models for in vivo testing of novel antidiabetic drugs.

The obesity and diabetes research will continue to benefit from the development of novel disease models. The use of transgenic or knock-out mice enables proof-of-concept studies on a target before beginning the drug development process. As an example the targeted inactivation of the DPPIV gene yielded healthy mice with improved insulin sensitivity and established DPPIV as a potential target for the therapy of type 2 diabetes [93]. These mutant mice are also of potential interest for discovering novel substrates of DPPIV as new drug targets. Peptidomics is the most potent technology to analyse proteolytic activity on a global scale. From numerous studies on diabetes mouse models there is now good reason to believe that obesity and diabetes are caused by several abnormalities in physiologic circuits regulated by hormones. The peptidomics technology enables researchers to identify new peptide hormones and alterations associated with the onset of a disease.

2.9 Profiling of Transcription Modulating Drugs

Petra Budde

In higher organisms the control of lipid and carbohydrate homoeostasis is dependent on the integration of signals from the central nervous system, traditional hormone systems as well as metabolites from lipids. Unlike transmembrane receptors for peptide hormones or cytokines, receptors binding small lipophilic ligands are located in the cytosol or nucleus and act as ligand inducible transcription factors. Following cloning of the classical steroid and thyroid hormone receptors, over 150 mammalian members of the so-called nuclear receptor superfamily have been identified [94]. Nuclear hormone receptors share an extensive homology and are thought to be evolutionarily derived from a common ancestor. This has led to the identification of new „orphan" receptors, whose ligands are yet to be discovered. Orphan receptors with pathophysiological activities represent potential drug targets. In the last few years, it has been increasingly realized that nuclear receptors are involved in key metabolic processes with great potential as targets for the treatment of significant diseases such as breast cancer, osteoporosis, coronary heart disease, and diabetes (Table 7). Collectively, these diseases represent a large market for prescription drugs worldwide [95].

Drug target	Drug name	Indication
Estrogen receptor (ER) Agonists and antagonists	Premarin (estrogen) Evista (raloxifene HCl) Nolvadex (tamoxifen citrate)	Menopause/osteoporosis Breast cancer
Peroxisome proliferator-activated receptor (PPARγ)	Avandia (rosiglitazone) Actos (pioglitazone)	Type 2 diabetes
Retinoic acid receptor (RXR)	Accutane (isotretinoin)	Acne
Glucocorticoid receptor (GR)	Flovent (fluticasone propionate) Advair (salmeterol) Pulmicort (budesonide) Flonase (fluticasone propionate)	Inflammation/asthma
Vitamin D receptor (VDR)	Calcitriol (1,25-dihydroxycholecalciferol)	Osteoporosis
Mineralocorticoid receptor (MR) Aldosterone antagonist	Aldactone (spironolactone)	Hypertension
Thyroid hormone receptor (TR)	Synthroid, Levoxyl Levothroid, Unithroid (levothyroxine)	Hyperthyroidism

Table 7: Top-selling drugs targeting transcriptional activators.

In some cases, specific ligands have been found for orphan nuclear receptors. For example the peroxisome proliferator activated receptor (PPAR) binds fatty acids with low affinity. Receptors that bind metabolic intermediates such as bile acids (farnesoid X receptor, FXR), and cholesterol intermediates (liver X receptor, LXR) are thought to act as metabolic sensors altering the expression of genes involved in energy metabolism and storage.

2.9.1 PPAR and metabolic diseases

It is now evident that obesity plays a primary role in the development of type 2 diabetes T2DM and is associated with elevated levels of free fatty acids (FFA). FFAs impair insulin signalling in muscle and can produce insulin resistance. Thus, lowering FFA levels would be beneficial in type 2 diabetes patients. Attempts to develop drugs lowering blood glucose levels have led to the development of the thiazolidinedione (TZD) drug class that significantly improves insulin sensitivity. Given the close relationship between disturbed lipid and glucose metabolism, the high therapeutic value of both TZD and lipid lowering fibrates was unmasked, identifying PPAR as their target.

PPARs include three individual genes with distinct cellular expression and biological functions. PPARα is expressed in muscle, liver, kidney and heart, regulates the fatty acid uptake and oxidation and is targeted by the fibrate class of drug. PPARδ is ubiquitous with highest expression in muscle. Its activation increases fatty acid oxidation in muscle making it another promising drug target. PPARγ is most abundantly expressed in adipose tissue and plays a critical role in adipocyte differentiation, lipid storage and glucose metabolism. Synthetic PPARγ agonists such as TZD are thought to result from direct actions on adipose tissue. However, the precise mechanism how TZD compounds improve insulin sensitivity is still elusive. Results obtained from gene expression studies suggest that the beneficial effects of TZD on liver, muscle, and pancreas are mostly secondary to PPARγ activation in adipocytes and mediated by (i) increased lipid uptake, (ii) decreased expression of proinflammatory cytokines, (iii) increased expression of adiponectin, and (iv) increased insulin action and glucose uptake. In addition to its action on adipocytes, as a lipid sensor PPARγ regulates macrophage functions at the vessel wall and reduces the formation of atherogenic foam cells. Therefore, TZDs exhibit additional therapeutic value for diabetic patients with increased risk of atherosclerosis. Fig. 49 (see page 98) summarises the physiological action of PPARγ agonists and affected genes.

The currently prescribed TZD compounds rosiglitazone and pioglitazone have proven to be efficacious as insulin sensitisers for the treatment of T2DM. Unfortunately, as full agonists these compounds promote enhanced adipogenesis. An undesired side effect is additional weight gain in patients which may result in diminished efficacy in already obese subjects. Questions remain over the long-term safety of TZD drugs following reports on potential side effects including cardiac hypertrophy, tumour and edema. Furthermore, troglitazone, launched in 1997 and the first drug in this class to reach the market, was later withdrawn due to hepatotoxic side effects. To retain the metabolic efficacy of PPARγ ligands and to reduce undesired side effects, substantial efforts are undertaken to improve PPARγ ligands. Different concepts have been developed in PPARγ ligand drug development.

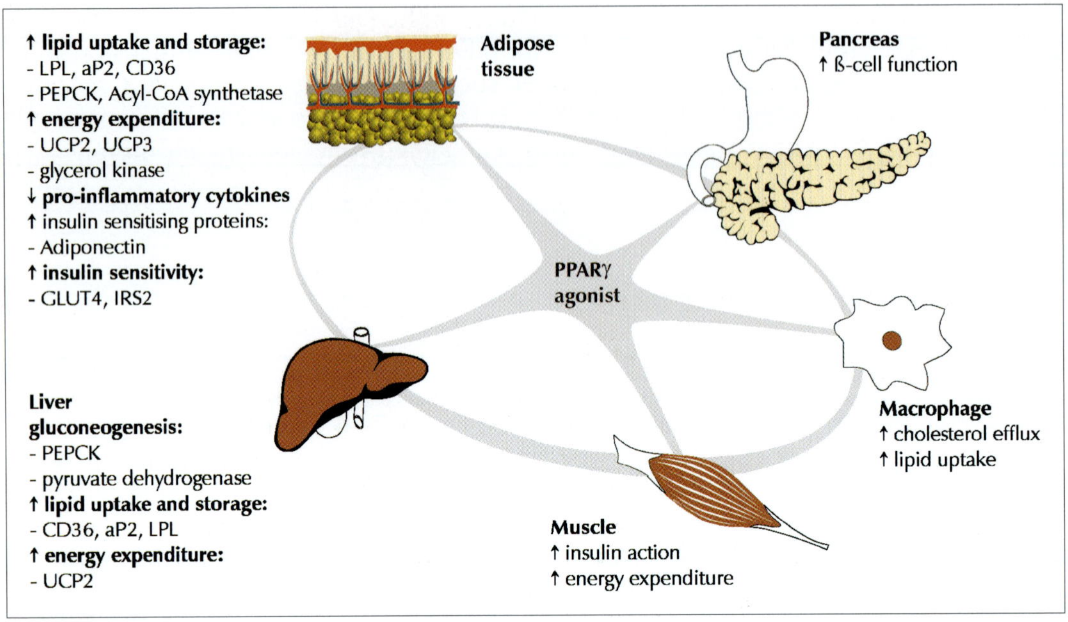

Fig. 49: Overview of genes affected by PPARγ activation in various tissues and organs.
Representative gene products of pertaining metabolic pathways and secreted mediators are shown: LPL, lipoprotein lipase; aP2, fatty acid binding protein; PEPCK, phosphoenolpyruvate carboxykinase; GLUT, glucose transporter; IRS, insulin receptor substrate; and uncoupling protein (UCP).

In analogy to the pioneering work to develop the first selective estrogen receptor modulator, tamoxifen, for the treatment of breast cancer, several selective PPARγ modulators were discovered that act as partial agonists or antagonists with promotor-, tissue- or cell type effects. Like other transcriptional regulators, PPARs exhibit a conserved modular structure: the N-terminal transactivation domain followed by a DNA binding region, a C-terminal ligand binding domain (LBD) and a motif that mediates the heterodimerisation with the retinoic acid receptor (RXR). The specificity of gene transcription is regulated by binding to a hexameric DNA sequence, the PPAR response element (PPRE). The concentration and types of ligand, specific coactivators and corepressors mediate the transcriptional activity in different tissues (Fig. 50).

MCC-555 is a novel TZD, presently in phase II clinical studies, that activates the LBD differently in different contexts, in part because of novel effects on coactivator recruitment [96]. Because the N-terminus of PPARγ is not required for activation by MCC-555 and corepressor recruitment is not stimulated, MCC-555 acts in a way distinctly different from the estrogen receptor partial agonist and antagonist tamoxifen. Comparison of the antidiabetic activity of MCC-555 with potent full agonists (troglitazone, pioglitazone and

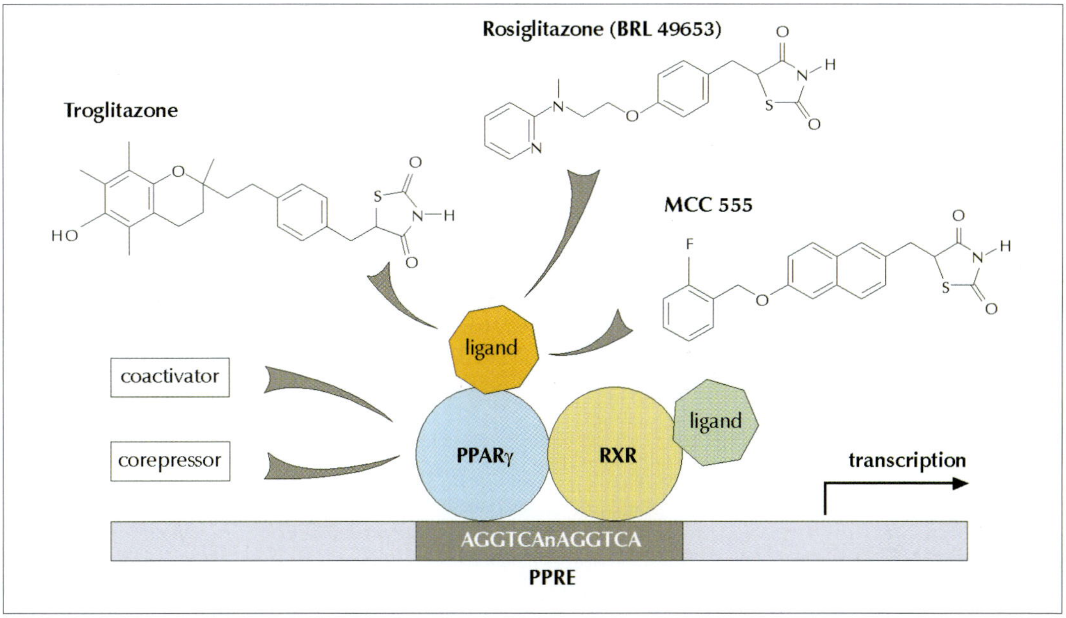

Fig. 50: Structure of PPARγ and agonists.

rosiglitazone) in obese KK-A^y mice revealed a three-fold lower ED_{25} for MCC-555 than that of rosiglitazone. Furthermore, MCC-555 improves metabolic status and insulin sensitivity in obese Zucker and diabetic ZDF rats. However, its binding affinity for PPARγ is less than 1/10 that of rosiglitazone. Similarly, MCC-555 induced adipocyte differentiaton, but as measured by the induction of the adipocyte specific aP2 gene the ED_{50} was approximately 10-fold greater for MCC-555 than for rosiglitazone.

2.9.2 Expression profiling approaches

Genes activated by PPARγ ligands have been screened extensively in 3T3-L1 adipocytes and adipose tissue. Gene expression profiling was carried out to examine whether novel non-TZD PPARγ partial agonists developed by Merck Research Laboratories produce a different expression pattern in 3T3-L1 adipocytes and adipose tissue compared to full agonists [97]. When 3T3-L1 adipocytes were treated with a 20-fold higher concentration of the respective ED_{50} all full agonists tested clustered together whereas the partial PPARγ agonist exhibited a distinct expression pattern. Several of the genes upregulated by full agonists involved lipid uptake and metabolism, such as lipoprotein lipase (LPL) and aP2, whereas the non-TZD partial agonists had little effect on their expression. Importantly, the effects on well-known adipokine such as adiponectin, TNFα or leptin mRNAs were similar.

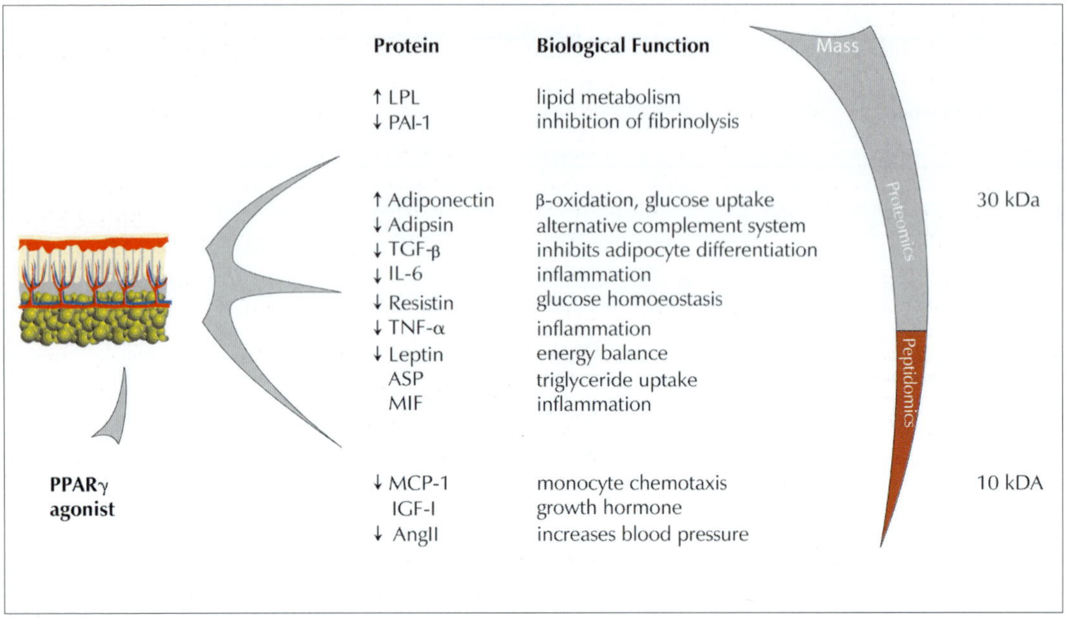

Fig. 51: Protein and peptide factors released by adipocytes.
Arrows indicate up- or downregulation by TZD. PAI-1, plasminogen activator inhibitor-1; TGF-β, transforming growth factor-β; IL-6, interleukin-6; TNF-α, tumour necrosis factor-α; ASP, acylation-stimulating protein; AngII, angiotensin II, MIF, macrophage inhibitory factor; MCP-1, macrophage chemoattractant protein-1; IGF-I, insulin-like growth factor-I.

Given the great therapeutic potential of TZDs as antidiabetic and anti-inflammatory drugs and the large number of adipokines secreted by adipocytes, continuing the study of TZDs actions on the protein and peptide level will provide further valuable information on the biochemical pathways implicated in the mode of action of novel PPARγ agonists. Similiar to transcriptomics, proteomics and peptidomics technologies can be applied to classify compounds and profile the action of a drug on a global scale. But unlike transcriptomics, proteomics and peptidomics are considered to provide measures of the final and functional products of the genes, the protein and peptides. Therefore, only integrating knowledge from parallel profiling techniques such as transcriptomics and proteomics will contribute to an in-depth understanding of the molecular mechanisms and physiological responses of transcription modulating drugs.

Adipose tissue itself secretes a number of bioactive proteins and peptides, termed adipokines, with autocrine/paracrine and endocrine function (Fig. 51). These adipokines influence diverse biological processes such as reproduction, energy homeostasis and immune function depending on the nutritional supply and the lipid stores available.

Obesity and in particular excess abdominal adipose tissue mass negatively influence the secretory profile of adipocytes and their capacity to store lipids properly. Adipose tissue secretion of proinflammatory cytokines, e.g. MCP-1, TNF-α and IL-6, is increased with obesity and insulin resistance and it is implicated in the development of atherosclerosis. A range of stimuli including insulin, glucocorticoids, sex steroids, TNF-α, growth hormone, FFAs and PPARγ agonists influence the expression of adipokines. Whereas the expression of proinflammatory cytokines decline with TZD treatment, the levels of adiponectin increase. Plasma adiponectin levels are strongly and inversely correlated with insulin resistance and atherosclerosis. Adiponectin exerts antidiabetic and antiatherogenic effects and is regarded as a major mediator of the beneficial TZD effect.

Several proteinases are also expressed in adipose tissue. These include renin, angiotensinogen converting enzyme (ACE) and other proteinases (chymase, cathepsin D and G) producing angiotensin II. Apart from its blood pressure regulating activity, angiotensin II promotes adipogenesis and decreases insulin-dependent glucose uptake. Blockade of the classical renin angiotensin system in patients with hypertension increases adiponectin concentrations [98]. Another proteolytic system involved in pathophysiology of obesity is the large family of matrix metalloproteinases (MMPs). Collectively, MMPs are able to cleave extracellular matrix (ECM) components and are induced during adipose tissue development and adipogenesis. Apart from their classical degradative activities, MMPs are able to release and process bioactive proteins and peptides with relevance to adipocyte biology, e.g. pro-TNF-α, MCP-1 or TGF-β.

2.9.3 Peptidomics profiling of TZD responsive small proteins and peptides

To accelerate the drug development process, proteomics and specifically peptidomics technologies are promising new approaches to discover novel protein and peptides markers as indicators of drug efficacy and adverse effects. One strategy to initiate the search for potential biomarkers that are indicative for the action of a certain TZD compound is to analyse adipose tissue where the protein and peptide concentration is presumably higher than in body fluids. An approach which profiles the expression of secreted protein and peptides appears to be most successful to facilitate the later detection of candidate proteins in plasma or serum.

An extensively used in vitro model is the murine 3T3-L1 preadipocyte line that can be converted to mature adipocytes upon hormonal stimulation which is easily monitored by the accumulation of large lipid droplets. Experiments were performed to identify secreted small proteins and peptides responsive to insulin signalling and regulated by PPARγ activation. This approach addresses the hypothesis that those peptides are mediators (or novel adipokines) of the insulin sensitising action of TZD compounds. Following a two-day treatment with troglitazone and acute insulin stimulation in various combinations, the conditioned medium was collected and processed by the peptidomics technology platform as described above (Fig. 52; see page 102). A typical resulting peptide display of 3T3-L1 supernatants consists of at least 5000 different signals in a mass range of 1–15 kDa. Using statistical data mining tools, several peptides were newly identified as

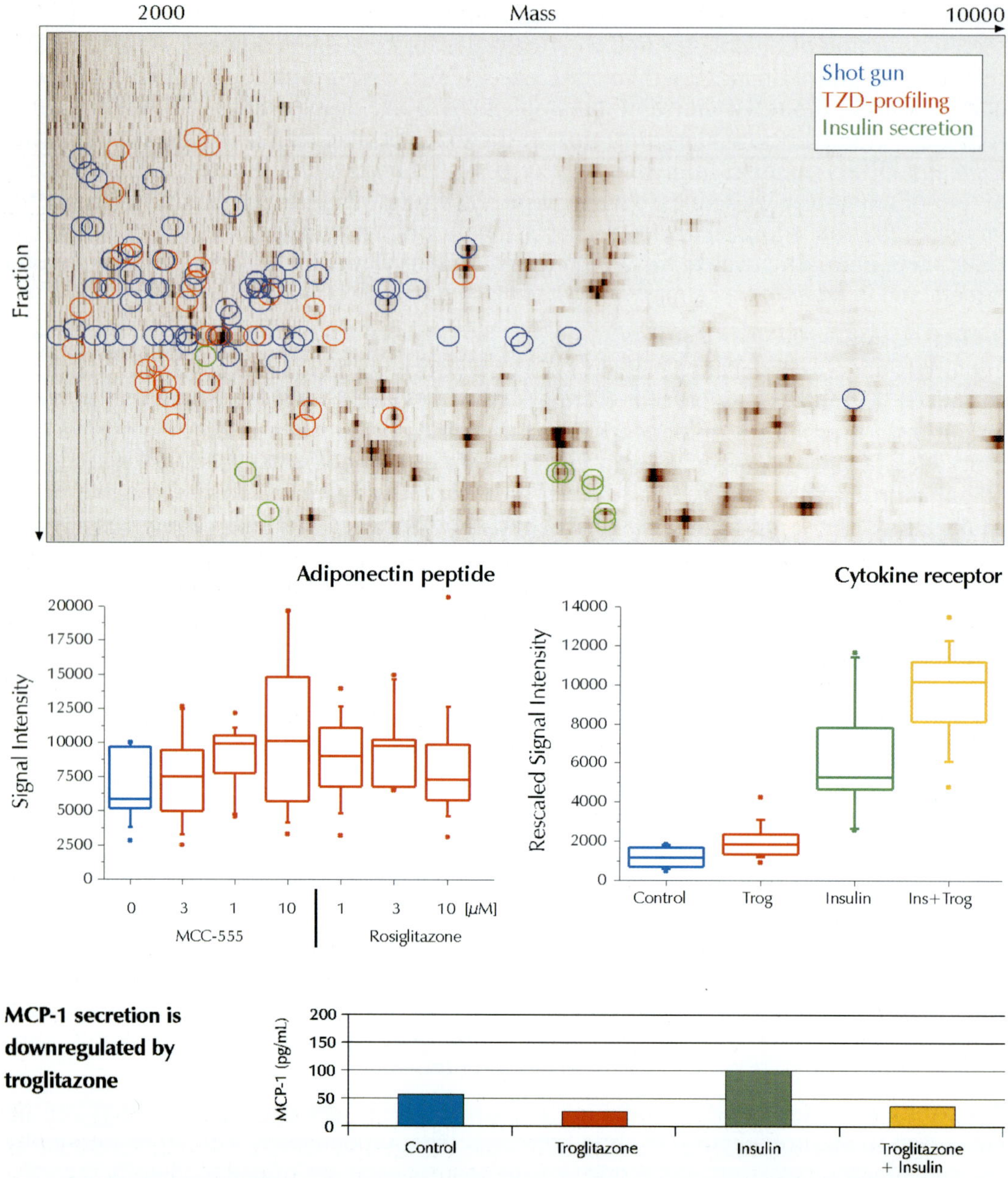

Fig. 52: Peptidomics technologies of adipocyte released peptides in response to TZD compounds.
3T3-L1 adipocytes were treated with vehicle (Control), MCC-555, troglitazone (Trog), rosiglitazone or a combination of troglitazone with and without insulin for 48 h, the supernatant was separated by HPLC (first dimension) and each fraction was separately analysed by MALDI-TOF MS to give the mass to charge ratio (m/z, second dimension). The resulting data were converted to a 2D graph. Both MCC-555 and rosiglitazone increased the expression of an adiponectin peptide. MCC-555 seems to be less potent than rosiglitazone.

adipocyte released factors that have been reported in other cell systems. The protein precursors of these peptides have been shown to play a role in cell differentiation and inflammatory processes. One of the newly discovered small proteins identified is a cytokine receptor released from the plasma membrane by proteolytic processing.

Another approach aimed to compare the potency of the full agonist rosiglitazone with the novel TZD MCC-555 that can act as a context specific partial agonist or antagonist. Depending on the assay used, the EC_{50} of MCC-555 is approximately 10-fold higher compared to rosiglitazone. 3T3-L1 adipocytes were treated for 48 h with 0, 1, 3 and 10 μM of MCC-555 and rosiglitazone. Peptides were analysed using non-parametric statistics to find peptides with concentration dependent increased or decreased signal intensities. Collectively, the majority of peptides were regulated concentration dependently by MCC-555, however with approximately 10-fold lower potency compared to rosiglitazone. These results suggest that for the majority of peptides released from 3T3-L1 adipocytes MCC-555 is functionally equal to rosiglitazone albeit less potent. Regarding the higher in vivo antidiabetic potency of MCC-555 it remains to be determined how this affects the expression of adipokines.

The TZD approach currently revealed > 100 regulated peptides. Among these the largest subset comprises peptides derived from larger protein precursors of known function. These can be clustered in groups including: (i) extracellular matrix and adhesion proteins, (ii) lipid uptake and metabolism proteins, (iii) secreted proteins, and (iv) ectodomains of transmembrane proteins. We also observed changes in the abundance of intracellular proteins involved in oxidative phosphorylation and glucose metabolism which correspond to the previously reported increase in mitochondria during adipogenesis. Of special interest is a novel adiponectin peptide that results from proteolytic processing of the precursor (Fig. 52). Serum adiponectin is found in several forms, one of which corresponds to the globular form with distinct metabolic activity and receptor binding profile compared to full-length adiponectin.

In summary, several novel peptides and small proteins derived from larger protein precursors were identified that have not been described previously. Our results strongly suggest that TZD compounds not only directly alter gene expression on the transcription level but also act indirectly in the post-translational pathway. This may either result in the generation of novel peptides with a putative biological function or an altered biological response of the remaining protein precursor.

2.10 Functional Peptidomics

Marco Jost, Nicolas Le Yondre, and Rüdiger Hess

2.10.1 Introduction

The discovery of bioactive peptides has always been an important task. One classical approach to identify such peptides is the combination of biotests with biochemical purification. Usually, separation of crude extracts from tissues or other biological sources into several fractions is performed by a series of liquid chromatography steps followed by the determination of bioactivity in these fractions, a procedure carried out in repetitive cycles until purity allows for sequence identification. Such methods have been successfully used for the identification of several bioactive peptides [99–101]. However, the final identification of the bioactive peptide with these methods is rather time consuming and needs large amounts of starting material. Here we describe a concept for the implementation of the differential peptide display technique into a functional peptidomic platform using the insulinoma cell line INS-1 as a model system. Functional peptidomics is defined as the combination of functional readouts with peptidomics data from the same sample, with the concept to quickly detect and prioritise certain peptides with a higher likelihood of functional relevance. Such a strategy might be helpful for scientists aiming to identify peptides with functional importance.

2.10.2 Why functional peptidomics?

In contrast to the static genome the expression pattern of proteins/peptides is much more versatile. It is therefore obvious that the information of the gene sequence alone will not be sufficient to understand cellular functions. Depending on the computational method used the number of protein coding genes is currently estimated to be in the range of 20,000–25,000 genes [102]. From this limited starting pool of proteins a much more complex proteome is created by splicing and other essential modifications which are temporally, spatially, and quantitatively regulated. One major influence on the proteome is given by the effect of proteolytic enzymes which degrade and modify proteins. Up to now 504 proteases have been identified in Homo sapiens according to the last release of the MEROPS database [103]. This class of enzymes plays an important role in different biological mechanisms like blood clotting, inflammation, and glucose homeostasis. One action of the proteases is the generation of bioactive peptides from larger precursors which then mediate the biological effect. A well studied example is the generation of insulin from its precursor molecule. In the beta-cells of the pancreas proinsulin is cleaved by the action of the proteases C2/C3 and the carboxypeptidase H in two peptides, the connecting peptide (C-peptide) and active insulin [103, 104]. Pathological processes like insulin resistance and hyperglycemia or certain drugs which lead to an increase in insulin secretion finally evoke an impairment in the insulin processing mechanism reflected by high levels of uncleaved proinsulin [105]. Thus, at any time point the composition of the peptidome in body fluids or single cells will vary dependent on the impact of primary and secondary factors. From the diversity of the proteome/peptidome it became clear that it is necessary to focus research on functionally important differences. This strategy allows to prioritise the overwhelming information available on functionally relevant peptides. Such investigations might include the analyses of cells treated with drugs or physiological stimuli and detecting important functional differences, e.g. by alterations in the composition of the cell supernatant. We tested such an approach by altering the glucose concentration in the culture medium and inhibiting prohormone processing in the insulinoma cell line INS-1.

2.10.3 Functional peptidomics using INS-1 cells

To verify the influence of a physiological challenge on the peptide pattern and identify bioactive peptides secreted by the INS-1 cells we treated these cells with different concentrations of glucose (2 and 10 mM), a known stimulator of insulin secretion [106]. Supernatants were collected and the samples analysed as displayed in Fig. 53 (see page 106). Differential peptide display was performed by loading the samples onto a reversed-phase HPLC column with subsequent MALDI-MS analyses. Using this approach we could detect a total of approx. 3000 peptides in the samples. It is obvious that this huge number of peptides does not allow quick identification of the bioactive peptides released from INS-1 cells.

In the next step we therefore measured bioactivity of the fractionized samples. As insulin is known to stimulate glucose uptake and inhibit lipolysis [107] we treated cultured fat cells with the fractionized INS-1 samples and measured changes in these parameters. As shown in Fig. 53 some fractions of INS-1 cells treated with the high concentration of glucose showed a stronger glucose uptake rate and blocked the release of free fatty acids into the supernatant. These fractions were selected for an additional reversed-phase HPLC step using a micro column. Changing the chromatographic conditions at this step (e.g. buffer, column size, gradient conditions) allows to further reduce the number of candidate peptides. Displays generated from these samples revealed approximately 20 signals per fraction corresponding to 1/10 of signals obtained from the original INS-1 supernatant. Again, glucose uptake of adipocytes was determined with these fractions and assigned to the mass spectrometric signals in the peptide display by a correlation of the elution behaviour of peptides (determined by their signal intensity) and the measured bioactivity. Using this approach two correlating m/z ratios were detected, with the first signal showing two maxima in bioactivity. This first signal was identified as rat insulin by MS/MS sequencing of the beta-chain. The second signal was identified as the insulin-1 precursor showing an increased signal intensity in the 10 mM glucose treated sample and a comparably weak effect on glucose uptake, as typically observed for the insulin precursor [108, 109].

The described utilization of functional peptidomics for the identification of bioactive peptides in the supernatant of glucose stimulated INS-1 cells should be regarded as a proof-of-concept application which has to be adopted to the more advanced scientific task to identify bioactive compounds where the molecular nature is unknown. This could

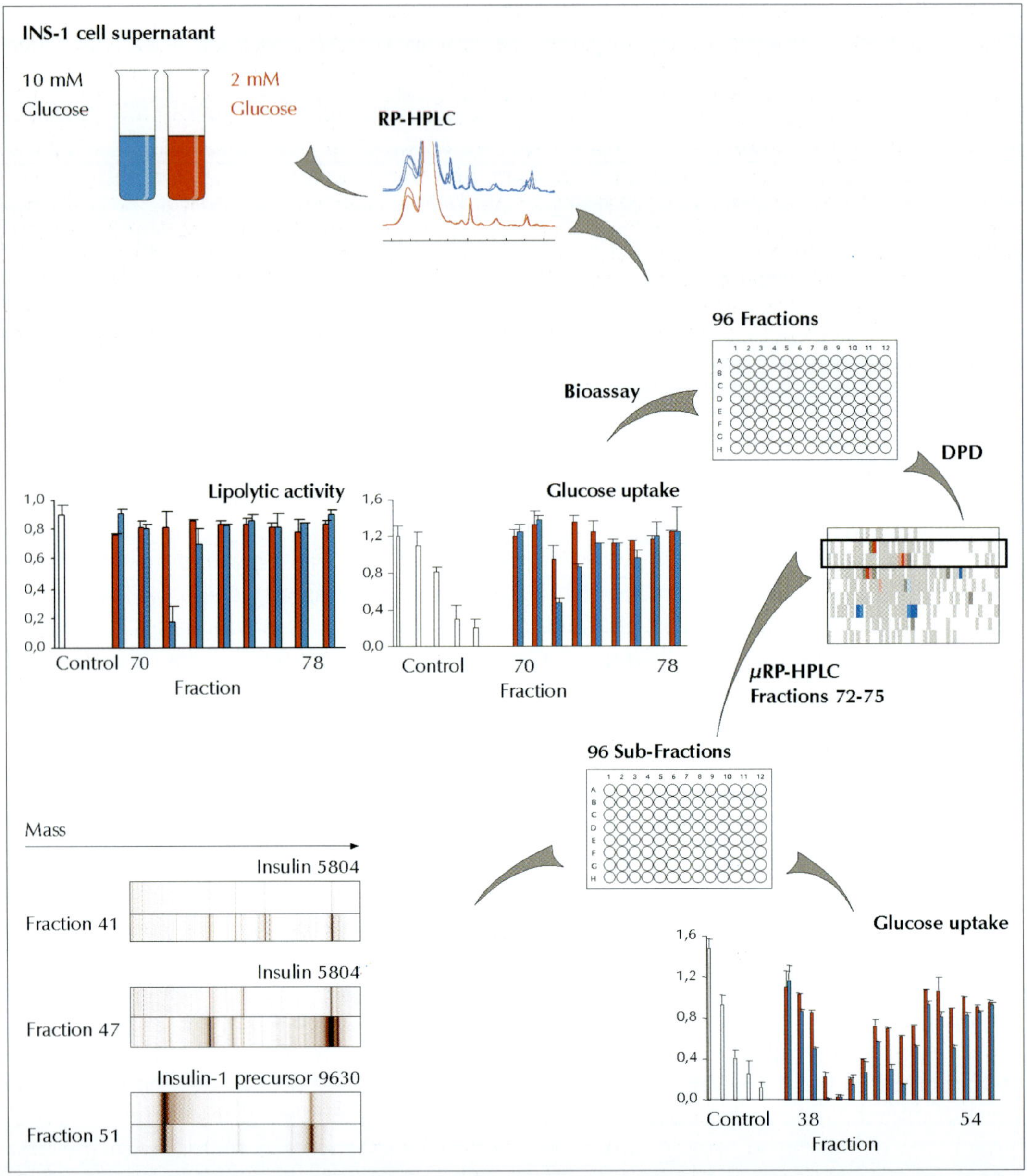

Fig. 53: Caption is shown on opposite page.

Fig. 53: Flow diagram of the employed strategy to identify bioactive peptides.
INS-1 cells were treated with 2 and 10 mM glucose and supernatants collected after 24 hours. An equivalent of 20 ml cell culture supernatant was loaded onto a RP-HPLC and peptides were separated in 96 fractions. 500 µl of cell culture supernatant was subjected to MALDI-MS. The converted mass spectra of all 96 fractions were combined resulting in a virtual two-dimensional display of peptide masses and elution times termed peptide display. Detection of differentially expressed peptides was achieved by calculation of subtractive peptide displays or correlation analysis (Differential Peptide Display) by referring to mass spectrometric data. In parallel stimulation of glucose uptake and inhibition of lipolysis by each fraction was measured in 3T3-L1 adipocytes. Bioactive fractions (Fr. 72-75) were selected and separated by means of µRP-HPLC in 96 sub-fractions (re-chromatography). We determined within these sub-fractions the rate of glucose uptake by adipocytes and performed a differential analyses between 2 mM and 10 mM stimulated INS-1 supernatants. In the fractions 41, 47, and 51 peptides were found to be increased by 10 mM glucose and these fractions led to an increased glucose uptake in cultured adipocytes. MS/MS sequencing identified these signals as insulin peptides and the insulin-1 precursor.

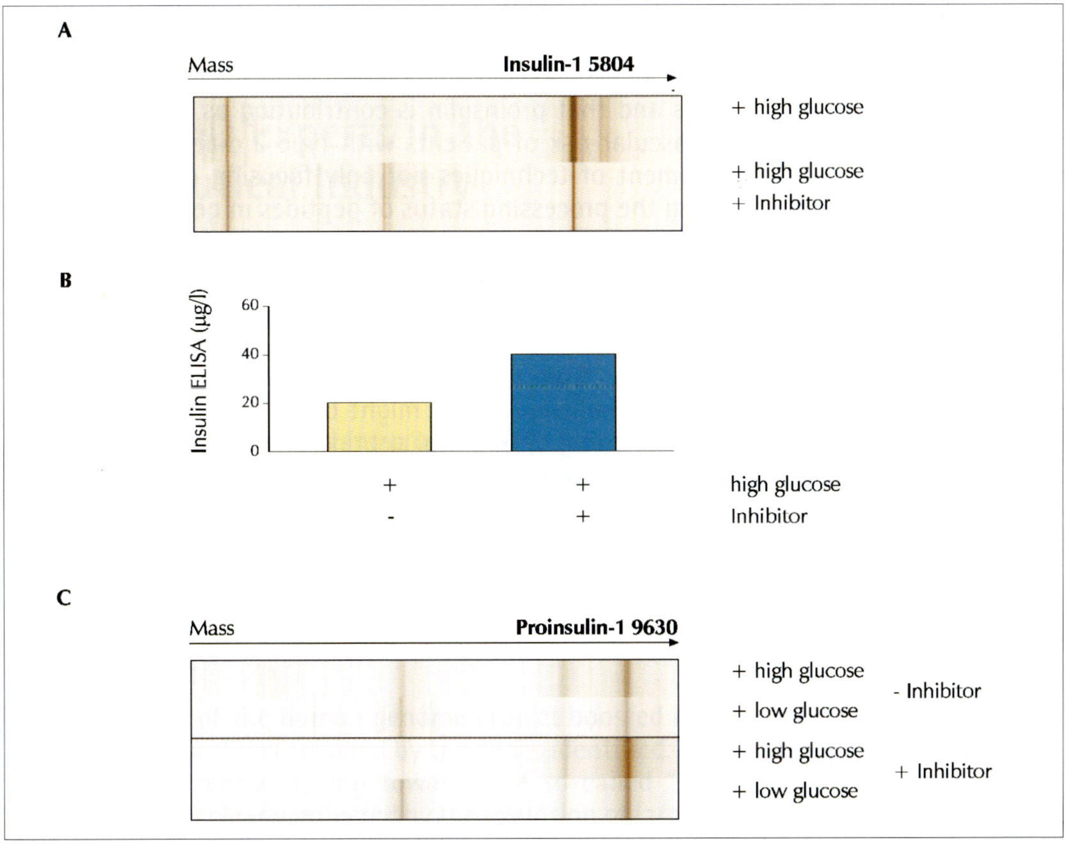

Fig. 54: Quantification of proinsulin and insulin-1 secretion.
INS-1 cells were treated with or without 100 µM of an inhibitor of prohormone processing (Dec-RVKR-CMK) for 24 hours. Then cells were stimulated with 10 mM glucose for 4 hours and supernatants collected for further analysis using DPD (A and C) and insulin ELISA (B).

Peptides are sequentially and selectively generated by a complex network of proteases to release multiple regulated metabolic functionalities. As such the world of peptides adds up to the extraordinary diversification from a single gene to complex functionalities. Within the continuous maturation-, activation-, and degradation cycle, any particular peptide structure and concentration reflects the particular metabolic processes involved.

Peptides have a paramount biological importance as biochemical messenger molecules organising the myriad regulatory processes maintaining the steady state of the human body. They function as hormones, neuropeptides, cytokines, enzyme inhibitors, and antimicrobial agents. However, due to technological limitations peptides have been neglected in most proteomic studies so far. The integrated analysis of the peptide content, which in analogy with the proteomics technology, aims at the simultaneous visualisation and identification of all peptides expressed in a cell or tissue, is a comparatively new technique [2] and the term peptidomics was introduced at the ABRF (Association of Biomolecular Research Facilities) conference in 2000 [1].

The 'one gene – one enzyme' paradigm and the concomitant notion that one gene or marker will be diagnostic of a disease has been replaced by a more nuanced understanding of the genesis of disease. With the exception of comparatively rare monogenetic disorders, most diseases are a consequence of complex alterations and there has been an increased realisation that a single marker is not sufficient for the accurate molecular diagnosis of disease, and that in many cases a single drug will not be sufficient to treat a disease. Thus, the measurement and characterisation of marker distribution patterns is pivotal in differentiating between different disease types and disease stages, and between normal and pathological conditions. The characterisation of peptidomes and their subsequent analysis from all kinds of samples reveals an in situ portrait of the complex dynamics of the proteome. In this way peptidomics may significantly contribute to the understanding of the human proteome both as a complementary and as a stand-alone tool. For drug research peptides are attractive in various ways: they are ideal markers to trace pathologic alterations, to monitor drug efficacy and adverse events, they may serve as drug candidates or drug targets, and they reflect the activity of proteases, which themselves play a crucial role as drug targets.

The importance of peptides for therapeutic applications became evident at the turn of the last century already when insulin as the first therapeutic peptide was used for treatment of diabetes. Today most drugs in use are small molecules, quite a number of which mimic the activity of peptides. The involvement of peptides in distinct disease areas either as drugs themselves or as target points at which drug therapy is directed is impressive, ranging from oncology via neurodegeneration, osteoporosis, blood pressure regulation, blood glucose and fat metabolism to fertility and immunology. Interestingly, peptides from other than human sources proved to be highly potent therapeutic lead compounds: antimicrobial peptides from animals and plants serve as templates for new therapeutic antibiotics, and peptide toxins from the venom of snakes, snails, and spiders are examined for their potential application in neurological, cardiovascular, and cancer indications.

Another advantageous feature of peptides is their ability to traverse between compartments of an organism. Consequently, many pathogenic processes can be reflected by characteristic pathogenic changes in peptide composition of these body fluids, suggesting that the outcome of peptide analyses will also have a direct impact on the diagnosis of many diseases.

A further important applicability of peptidomics targets the efficiency of the drug development process itself. The technology driven acceleration of identification of drug targets and generation of new drug candidates has created characteristic bottlenecks downstream in drug development. One of these arises from the necessity to obtain proof-of-concept new drug candidates in humans as early as possible. Consequently, increasing pressure is arising to integrate "-omics" approaches in a way that may introduce a boost to drug development [110]. However, the availability of proof-of-concept trials is greatly dependent on the availability of new markers for drug efficacy and safety, which need to be easily accessible in body fluids such as serum or urine to guarantee the possibility for frequent monitoring. Peptides are an excellent tool for these approaches and the peptidomics technology may allow discriminating between peptide profiles reflecting physiological/adaptive responses, and changes related to pathology and toxicology.

3.1.2 Objectives

Peptidomics has a great potential to become an important tool in future pharmaceutical development. Its contributions to drug development have advanced within comparatively short time with extensive medical applications being developed by an increasing number of players in academia, biotechnology, and the pharmaceutical industry. Nevertheless compared to genomics and proteomics, peptidomics appears to be not yet fully established as a stand-alone technology. Few scientific papers deal with peptidomics alone and unlike the genomics- and proteomics approaches, whose value for pharmaceutical development has been discussed in comprehensive scientific reviews, there is only little awareness yet of the impact of peptides on drug development. We therefore wanted to determine the current role and future perspectives of peptidomics as perceived by the pharmaceutical industry. In a comprehensive electronic inquiry we asked opinion leaders in R&D from global pharmaceutical companies, which are actively involved in peptidomics research, to estimate the value of the peptidomics approach for the industry.

The primary goal of the study was to obtain expert analyses of the current and future impact of peptidomics on drug development. The central focus of the survey was on the significance of the technology for diagnostic, therapeutic, and toxicological approaches in seven major indications and on the estimated time frames in which peptidomics may gain importance for the industry. In addition respondents were asked to supply text responses regarding technological pros and cons, and future technological challenges. Further data collected include the interest in collaboration with biotech companies, and expected investments for peptidomics/proteomics approaches.

3.2 Methods

The assessment was performed as a 54-item electronic inquiry among R&D experts from global researching pharmaceutical companies. The inquiry included a mixture of quantitative and qualitative questions. Data were statistically analysed by SPSS.

Senior managers in R&D departments of 32 researching pharmaceutical companies with assumed peptidomics activities, which are based in Europe, Japan, and the USA were approached and asked to participate in an online inquiry to assess the importance of peptidomics for pharmaceutical drug development. Participants were offered a detailed report of the study outcome. The study was conducted in 2004; duration of the inquiry (time from first questionnaire completed to last questionnaire completed) was 3 months.

3.3 Results

3.3.1 Responder rate

Of the 32 global pharmaceutical companies approached, 30 reported to be actively involved in peptidomics. In 9 (30%) of the firms with peptidomics activities the company policy prohibited participation, because the required information was considered too sensitive to be communicated. The remaining 21 companies (70% of the companies with peptidomics activities) participated in the inquiry (Fig. 55); a total of 25 experts of these companies responded to the inquiry.

3.3.2 Participants

The 21 participating global pharmaceutical companies included 11 European, 7 US-American, and 3 Japanese companies (Fig. 56; see page 114).

Quite a number of the participating companies have already established separate R&D departments dealing with "-omics" technologies. In the remaining companies, these experts either held general strategic R&D positions or were involved with drug safety or lead compound development, respectively. Specialisation and position of the 25 participants were as follows: head of genomics, proteomics, or trinomics (7), head of toxicology (5), head of R&D (2), head of strategic research (3), vice president (1), senior director of science development (1), head of biomarket development (1), head of biotechnology (1), head of world-wide chemistry (1), head of molecular biology and chemistry (1), head of lead discovery technologies (1), director of cancer infection bioscience (1).

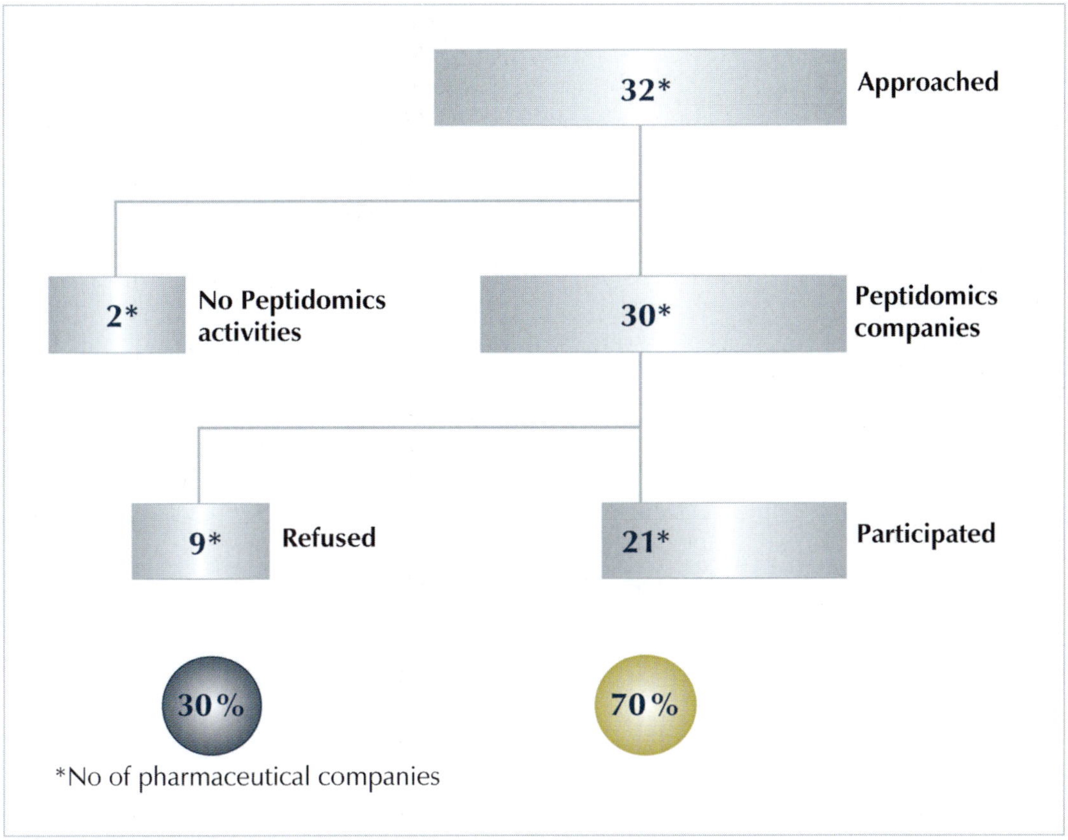

Fig. 55: 70% of the 'Peptidomics companies' participated in the Inquiry.

3.3.3 Peptidomics in various areas of drug development

Most respondents considered the application of peptidomics as 'likely' or 'very likely' in all areas of drug development investigated. Medical diagnostics appears to be the field with the highest potential for peptidomics, 96% of the participants chose 'likely' or 'very likely', followed by prediction of therapeutic success (88%), toxicology (68%) and development of lead compounds (64%) (Fig. 57; see page 114).

Abbott (3)*	Chiron Behring (1)	Roche (1)
Altana Pharma (2)	Eisai (1)	Sankyo Pharma (1)
Amylin Pharmaceuticals (1)	Genzyme (1)	Sanofi Synthelabo (1)
AstraZeneca (1)	Johnson & Johnson (1)	Schering (1)
Aventis (1)	Merck & Co (1)	Serono Pharma (1)
Bayer (1)	Novartis (2)	Takeda (1)
Boehringer (1)	Pfizer (1)	Tibotec (1)

*No of participants

Fig. 56: 25 Experts from 21 companies participated in the inquiry.

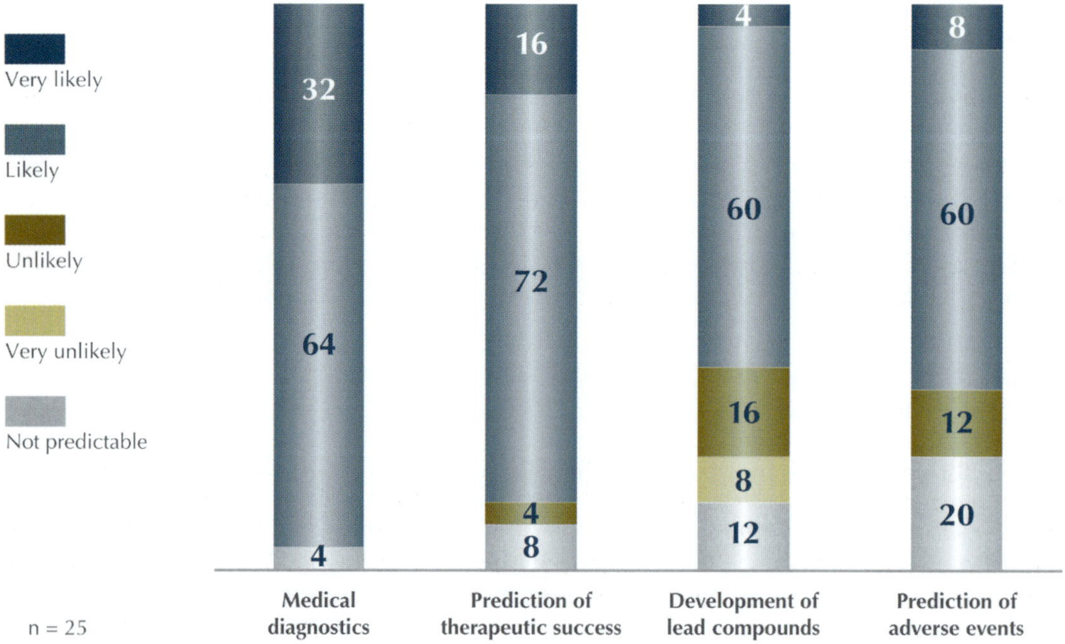

Fig. 57: Application of peptide biomarkers in different areas of drug development (%).

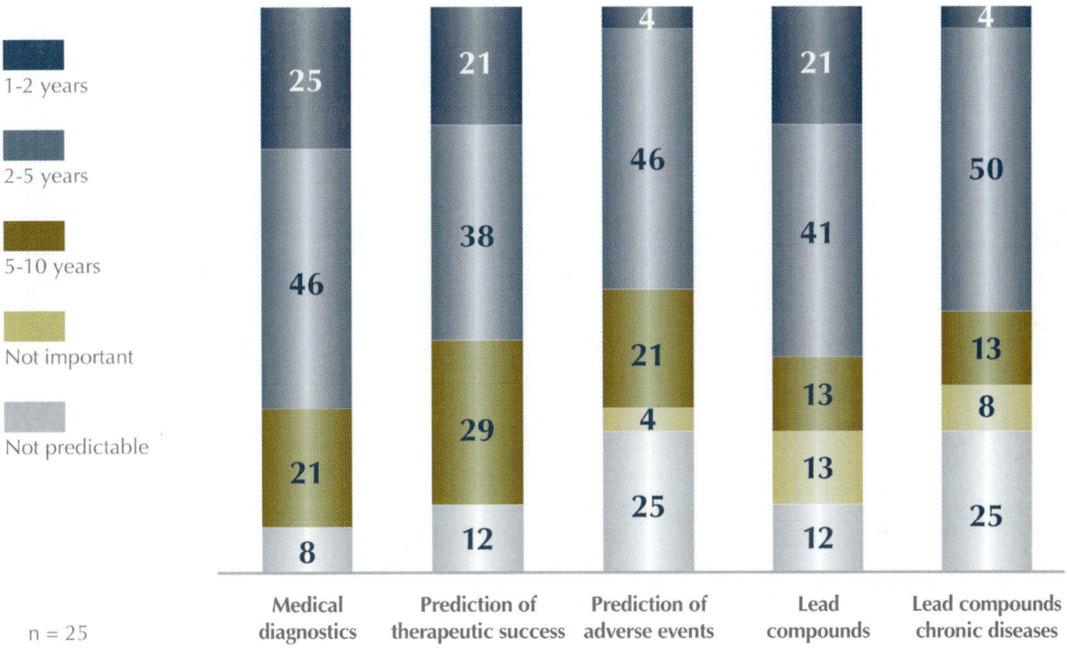

Fig. 58: Time frame for application of Peptidomics in different areas (%).

3.3.4 Time frames

Regarding the time frame within which peptidomics may become important in different areas of drug development, most companies reported that it will play an important role in all fields of drug development within the next 5 years. Diagnostics is the field that will most likely be infiltrated by peptidomics soon, 71% of the respondents predicting a time frame of 1–5 years, followed by 62% for development of lead compounds, 59% for prediction of therapeutic success, 54% for development of lead compounds for chronic diseases, and 50% for prediction of adverse events (Fig. 58).

3.3.5 Diagnostics

Regarding the likelihood of a diagnostical application of peptidomics in major indications, oncology was considered the most important indication for peptidomics by most respondents (88% chose 'likely' or 'very likely') followed by cardiovascular diseases (84%), metabolic diseases (76%), neurodegenerative diseases (72%), infectious diseases (44%) and respiratory diseases (36%). Respiratory diseases was the only indication in which 'unlikely' and 'very unlikely' was chosen by slightly more responders (40%) than 'likely' or 'very likely' (34%) (Fig. 59; see page 116).

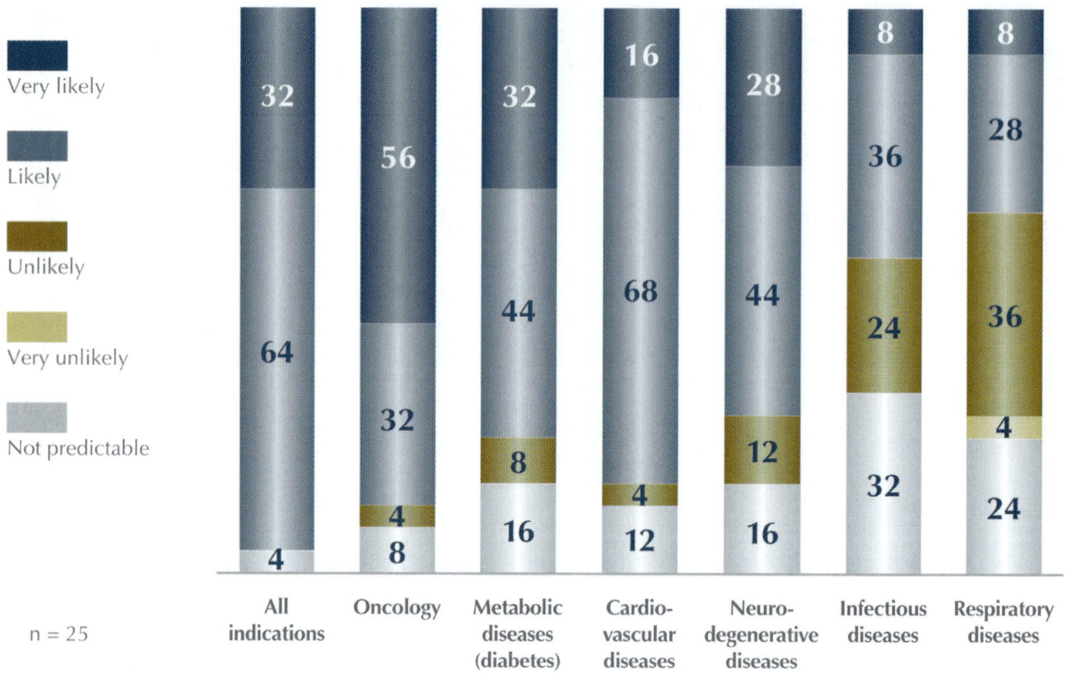

Fig. 59: Diagnostic application of peptide biomarkers (%).

3.3.6 Prediction of therapeutic success

For prediction of therapeutic success and the development of lead compounds, the reported importance of peptidomics for individual indications was very similar to that reported for diagnostics. For both fields of drug development, oncology was again considered the most important indication, while the predicted importance of respiratory diseases was low. For prediction of therapeutic success the reported frequencies of 'likely' and 'very likely' were 84% for oncology, 76% for metabolic diseases, 64% for cardiovascular diseases, 64% for neurodegenerative diseases, 44% for infectious diseases, and 32% for respiratory diseases (Fig. 60).

3.3.7 Development of lead compounds

For the development of lead compounds the corresponding rates were 64% for oncology, 64% for metabolic diseases, 52% for cardiovascular diseases, 52% for neurodegenerative diseases, 36% for infectious diseases, and 28% for respiratory diseases (Fig. 61).

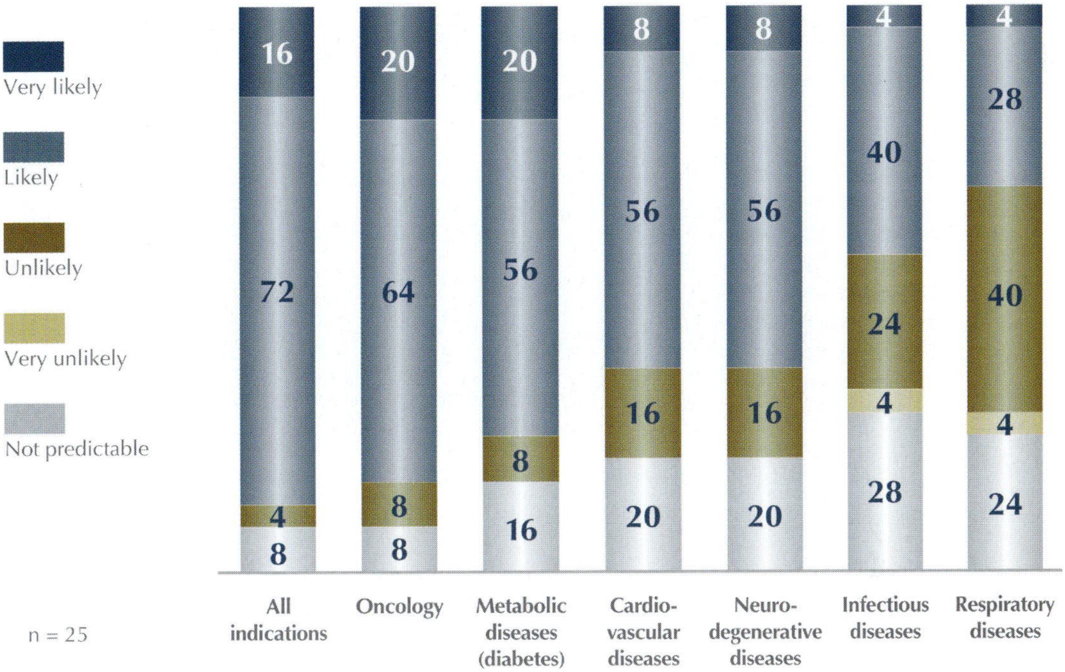

Fig. 60: Peptide biomarkers for prediction of therapeutic success (%).

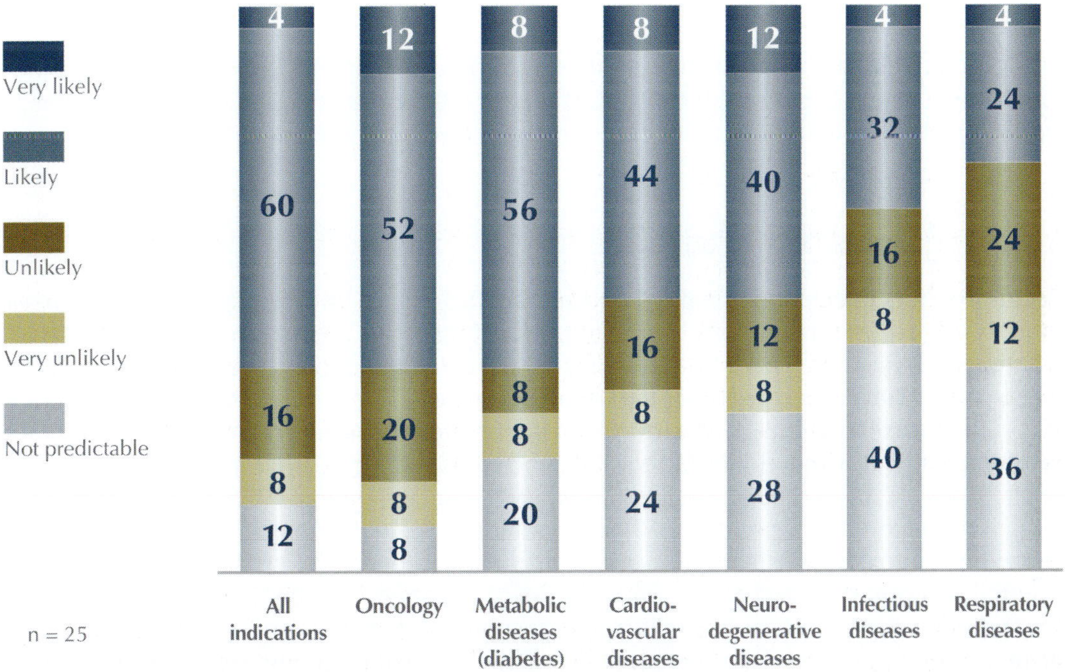

Fig. 61: Peptide biomarkers for the development of lead compounds (%).

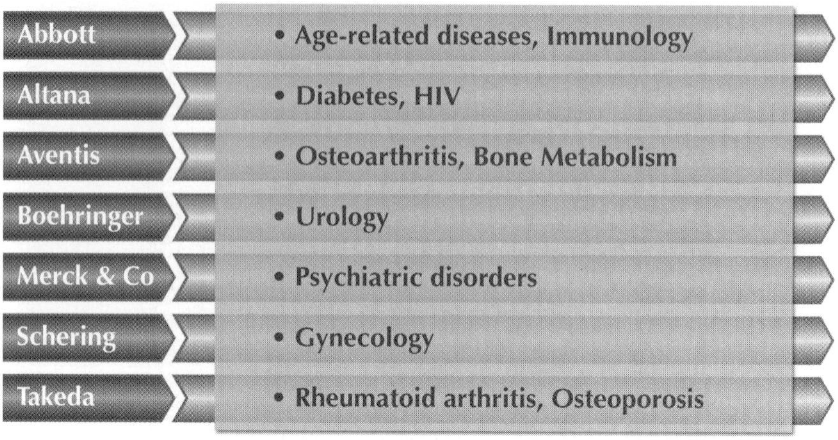

Fig. 62: Additional indications of interest.

3.3.8 Additional indications

In addition to the major indications mentioned above, participants were asked to add other indications, which they considered important for a potential application of peptidomics. Fig. 62 shows the additional fields of interest as reported by seven companies.

3.3.9 Molecular toxicology

Regarding the fairly new field of molecular toxicology, most respondents reported that peptide biomarkers will provide useful tools for prediction of adverse drug reactions in the near future; 68% of the participants chose 'likely' or 'very likely' when asked how important peptide biomarkers will be within the next 2-5 years (Fig. 63). Correspondingly, 52% of the respondents reported that the technology of peptidomics will become important for molecular toxicology within the next 2-5 years; 24% of the respondents predicted that the technology will impact this field within the next 5-10 years (Fig. 63). Compared to other technologies that play a role in molecular toxicology, peptidomics is considered to be of lower importance; 68% of respondents reported that the importance of peptidomics will be 'likely' or 'very likely'; for the other technologies the equivalent responder rates were much higher, i.e. 88% for bioinformatics, 88% for metabonomics, 84% for genomics, and 84% for proteomics (Fig. 63).

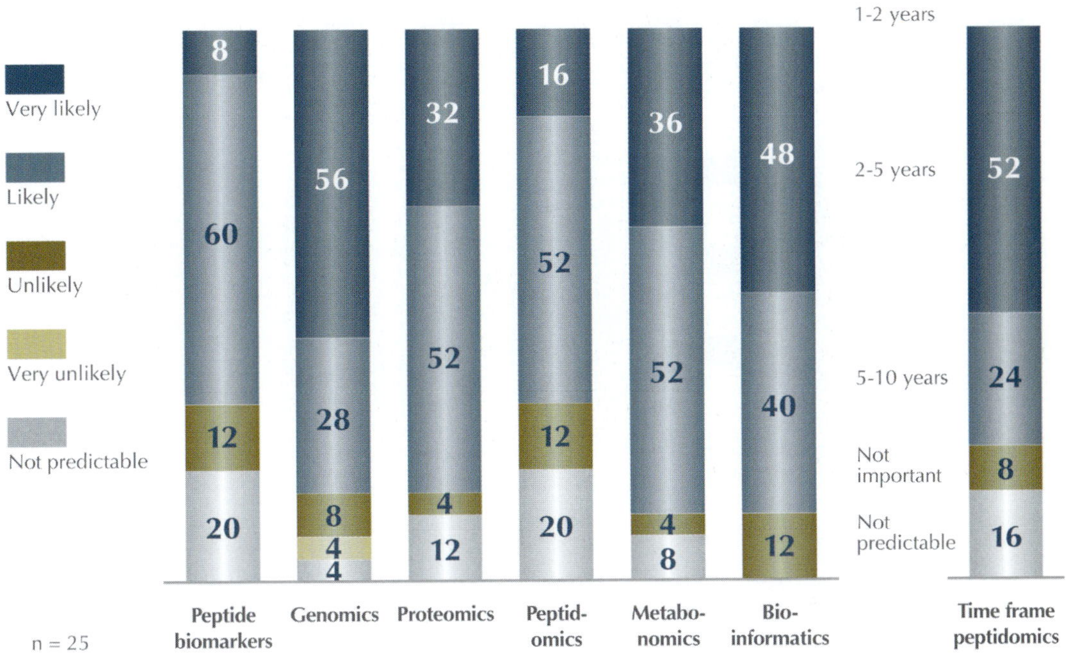

Fig. 63: Impact of various technologies on drug development.

3.3.10 Coopcration with biotcch companics

Most pharmaceutical companies reported that they are interested in collaborating with biotech companies regarding bioinformatics tools for peptidomics. More than 80% of the respondents reported that it was 'likely' or 'very likely' that they will seek collaboration within the next 1-5 years (Fig. 64); 42% of the respondents reported that only parts of larger projects will be sourced out to biotech companies, whereas 58% intend to source out both, entire projects as well as parts of a project (Fig. 64; see page 120).

3.3.11 Nature of collaboration

We also asked the participants to specify the nature of applications they intend to source out or conduct in-house. The results show that extent and type of applications performed in-house versus the applications that will likely be sourced out vary among companies. While a small company such as Tibotec will source out all peptidomics activities, Roche intends to perform most of the applications in-house. In Fig. 65 (see page 121) a detailed list of all responses is depicted.

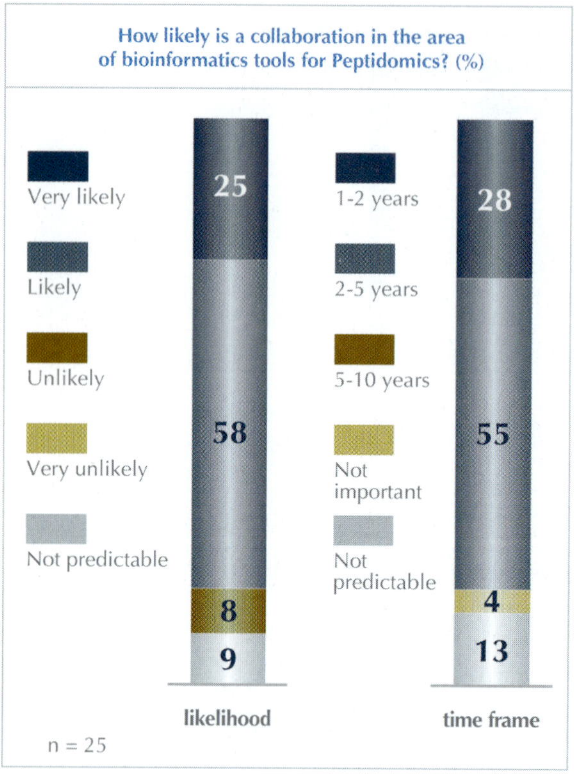

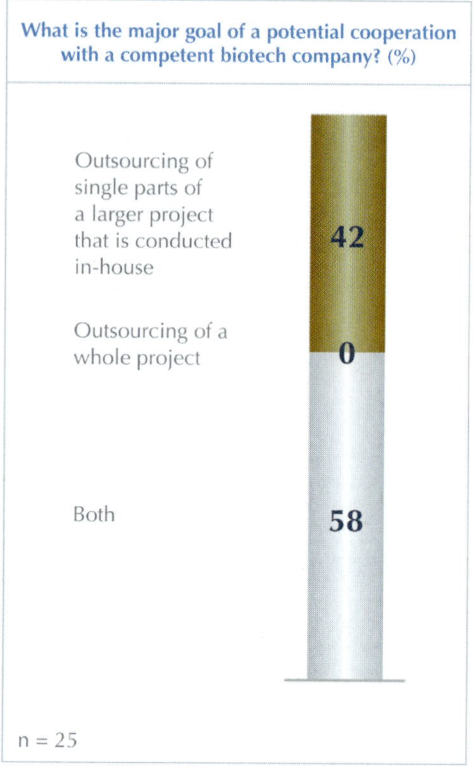

Fig. 64: Cooperation with biotech companies (%).

3.3.12 Technology assessment

In a further qualitative set of questions we asked the participants to describe the advantages and disadvantages of peptidomics. Regarding the advantages, respondents stressed the importance of new peptide biomarkers, which are easily accessible in body fluids. A number of respondents also considered the technology to be easier, faster and more easily reproducible than proteomics. Individual responses included:

Advantages of peptidomics

- Peptides are more readily accessible through body fluids (serum/plasma, CSF, urine) than full length proteins; peptides reflect the expression and modulation of their full length originators
- Easy blood tests
- Applicability to biofluids, i.e. non-invasive

	In-house	Source out
Abbott	Tox profiling, pred. of side effects, diagnostics	Target finding, validation efforts, based on peptide signatures, evaluation of disease biomarkers
Altana	Lead compound optimization, research decisions	Biomarker screening, developmental activities
AstraZeneca	IP sensitive experiments	Technology development, clinical studies
Aventis	Biomarkers for lead finding, toxicity pred.	Diagnostic biomarker, efficacy biomarker
Bayer	Evaluation part	Technical part
Boehringer	Compound related readouts	Disease-related marker discovery
Chiron	Chips	Epitope mapping
Eisai	Identifying biomarkers	
Genzyme		If any on a case by case basis for ident. of markers for patient stratification or pharmacodynamic efficacy
Tibotec	None	Target discovery, mechanistic toxicology
J&J	Predictive toxicity screening	Mechanistic or investigative toxicology studies
Merck & Co	High throughput screening	Initial discovery
Novartis	Proof of concept – and technical development studies	Routine/Mass Analysis
Pfizer	Assay development	Separate and identify peptides
Roche	Mostly in-house	Only peaks will be outsourced

Fig. 65: In-house and outsourced Peptidomics activities.

- Relevant, if available, serum markers are easy to access
- Tailored clinical trials (fewer patients may be needed to demonstrate efficacy and safety)
- Possibility to provide biomarkers for efficacy and safety; identification of "susceptible" and "at risk" patients
- Source of new biomarkers
- Relatively easy technology; analysis could be performed via image analysis; fits into the gap which is not filled by other technologies, focused characterisation

- Fast, assay development (AQUA) relatively straightforward
- Fast readout, relatively simple to perform
- Reproducibility (compared to proteomics)
- Provides more complete coverage of proteomic changes
- Subset proteome
- New has potential

Major objections concerned the relative lack of experience with the technology of peptidomics compared to genomics and proteomics. Also, it was pointed out that peptidomics – just as conventional proteomics techniques – reflects only one part of the whole proteome and it was indicated that the technology should be applied in combination with the other „-omics" technologies. Individual responses included:

Disadvantages of peptidomics

- Too many open questions on relevance of "biomarkers" and acceptance by agencies
- More technological development is needed and the wealth of data accumulated needs to be effectively processed, stored and made publically available
- First a marker should be found
- New; may be difficult to develop the diagnostic for small peptides
- Low knowledge base
- Needs experts and expensive equipment, difficulties in interpretation today
- High cost
- Feasibility and HT application of technology
- Peptides reflect only the low MW part of the proteome. Major part is proteolytically generated which may be or may not be disease related
- Hard to find receptors, hard to find non-peptidergic agonist/antagonist
- Poorly defined determinants peptide purification technology.
- Only a partial view of the proteome, low sensitivity (same problem as proteomics)
- No direct relationship to genes
- Should not be used alone (combination with other technologies required)

In view of the respondents the next steps in peptidomics need to focus on technological progress, the integration of associated tools such as bioinformatics for data interpretation, and further validation of the technology itself for its application in various areas of drug development. Individual responses included:

Next steps in proteomics

- Novel, and highly sensitive technologies and possibilities to include analysis of secondary modulation (phosphorylation, glycosylation, glycation, etc.), automation, higher throughput, demonstration of relevance of peptides as biomarkers

- Easiness to handle in order to become a valid diagnostic tool in hospitals in the future; data archives, historical references
- Understanding of the plethora of peaks, measurement of discrete analytes
- Generate knowledge how measured peptides relate to efficacy or toxicity; large validation programmes may be needed
- Most important issue in peptidomics is the quantitative comparison of peptide containing mixtures in a differential peptide/protein display for marker discovery
- Bioinformatics
- Integration into existing platforms; data integration and bioinformatics
- Interpretation of peptide profiling data
- Tools to incorporate across a broad range of technology platforms including bioinformatics
- Examples of success resulting in decreased cost or time of product development
- Validation identification capacity pool of endogenous peptides (what % existing peptides can be picked up, what are limiting constraints, etc.), efficient quantitation for sample to sample comparison
- Deeper mechanistic understanding of the function of those peptides – easy, cheap and robust analystics, i.e. in contrast to 2D gels
- Follow-on assay development (e.g. AQUA); bioinformatics / systems biology tools to understand data in the context of a living organism / disease
- Prefractionation to increase sensitivity
- Sensitivity, isolation method

3.3.13 Budget

Some companies were able to point out their estimated investment for peptidomics within the next five years. They also specified to which degree individual areas of drug development are covered by this investment and what percentage of the total investment will be spent for external cooperation. Among the 5 companies responding to this set of questions, there seems to be no common preference regarding the field of interest; instead, different companies seem to focus on different areas of drug development. Similarly, the percentage of the investments that will be spent for collaborations differs largely between companies, ranging from 30% to 90% (Fig. 66; see page 124).

Regarding the investments in the field of proteomics, Roche published that they will spend 100 million CHF within the next few years for proteomics research activities, which will link proteomics research in their Pharmaceuticals and Diagnostics Divisions. Johnson & Johnson estimated their investments for proteomics within the next 5 years to be 1.5 million USD and Sankyo reported to invest about 100,000 USD for research in proteomics within this time frame.

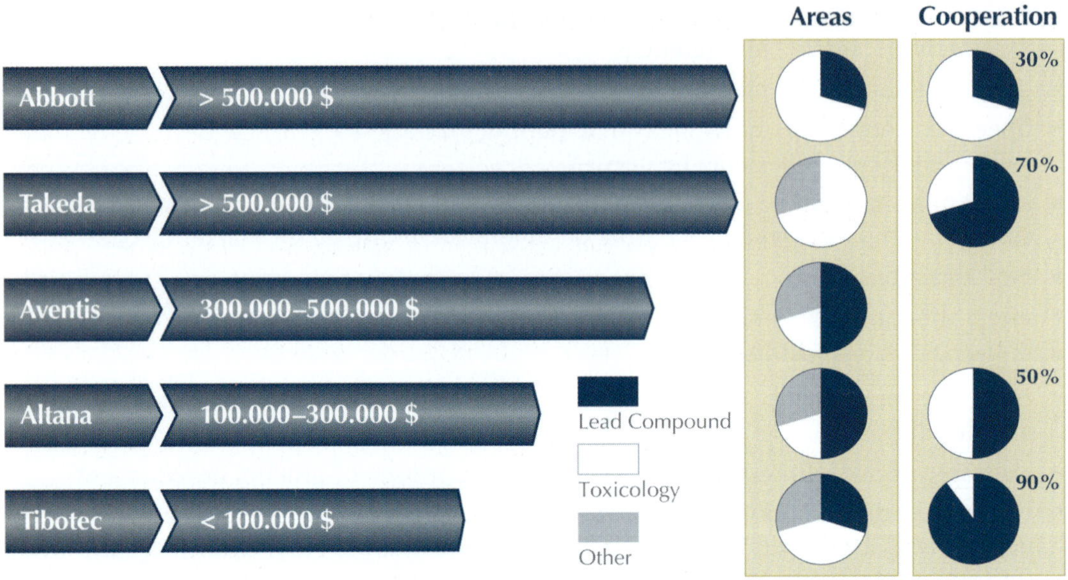

Fig. 66: Investments for Peptidomics within the next 5 years.

3.4 Conclusion

3.4.1 Responder rate

With few exceptions the response to the inquiry was extremely positive. Most specialists of R&D departments we approached were highly interested in the study and its outcome, even in those cases where the company policy prohibited participation. Correspondingly, the acceptance of the investigation was reflected by a high responder rate; 25 senior managers from 21 pharmaceutical companies unhesitatingly expressed their willingness to participate. Peptidomics is a novel technology only applied by pharmaceutical companies with a clear commitment to and capacity for innovative drug development. Of the 32 global companies we approached, 30 reported that they are actively involved in peptidomics research, while 2 companies were not active in this field. The 21 participating companies represent 70% of the global pharmaceutical companies with activities in peptidomics with their headquarters in Europe, USA, and Japan. The study outcome can therefore be considered as representative for the current view of R&D experts of innovative global pharmaceutical companies.

3.4.2 Peptidomics in various areas of drug development

According to the judgment of the pharmaceutical R&D senior managers, peptidomics will play a significant role in drug development in all major fields of drug development within the next 5 years. The majority of the respondents predicted that the technology will impact medical diagnostics, prediction of therapeutic success, lead compound development, and molecular toxicology. Especially medical diagnostics was indicated by 96% of the respondents to be an important field of application. This may well reflect the physiological key role of peptides making them prone to be involved in pathological processes in a variety of medical indications. Also, diagnostics is frequently the first area in medicine to be infiltrated by novel technologies, peptidomics being obviously one example of this phenomenon. Consequently, only 4% of the respondents considered the potential impact of peptidomics on diagnostics as unpredictable, whereas for prediction of therapeutic success, development of lead compounds, and prediction of adverse events, the experts were less certain; 8%, 12% and 20% chose unpredictable in these areas, respectively. Especially for the comparatively novel area of molecular toxicology, the impact of peptidomics seems to be difficult to predict. However, this does not necessarily mean that peptides may not eventually increase in importance as molecular toxicology matures. There is increasing focus on toxicology markers particularly in the preclinical area and a recent review predicted that molecular toxicology will likely prove one of the most important applications of proteomics [112].

3.4.3 Peptide therapeutics

Although peptides have a high potential to be used as drugs, a drawback of peptide therapeutics is their rapid degradation after ingestion, and that is why they usually have to be administered by injection. However, currently the pharmaceutical industry is developing alternative intranasal, enteral, and inhalative administrations [113, 114]. This limitation may have caused 24% of the responders to predict that for the development of lead compounds, the importance of peptidomics is unlikely or very unlikely and 13% predicted that this field will not be important for peptidomics within the next 10 years. Compared to other compound classes peptide therapeutics tended to have a negative image in the industry in the past. Yet it often proved difficult to find adequate molecular substitutes – the most prominent example being insulin. Interestingly, our investigation shows that the majority of experts (64%) consider the importance of peptidomics in lead compound development as likely or very likely and 62% predict that the technology will become important in this field within the next 5 years. This clearly indicates that peptide therapeutics and/or peptidomimetic approaches for lead compound development are perceived much more favourably by the pharmaceutical industry than it may have been expected.

This change in view is also reflected by current pharmaceutical pipelines. In 2003 the global therapeutic peptide market amounted to 1 billion USD and currently more than 40 peptide based products are commercially available with 6 in the registration process. In Europe, about 4 to 6 peptide based products are in the market, with 100 in the clinical stage and 150 in advanced pre-clinical phases. Peptides used in drug formulation and clinical trials account for nearly 93% of the European therapeutic peptides market with R&D comprising the remainder [115]. Examples for peptide drugs in use are insulin, parathyroid hormone (PTH), brain natriuretic peptide (BNP), calcitonin, antimicrobial peptides, protease inhibitors, and growth factors; numerous new chemical entities and generics are set to expand the market in coming years.

3.4.4 Biomarkers

The most preferential application of peptidomics is clearly the identification and validation of biomarkers. Physiological and pathological alterations are reflected by characteristic alterations in the proteome. Molecular characteristics that prove to be correlated to normal or pathological processes, or pharmacological responses to therapeutic intervention, may be used as biomarkers indicative for these processes. Biomarkers offer a widespread applicability in medicine and drug development. They serve as diagnostic tools, as indicators of drug efficacy and adverse events, and last not least versatile peptide expression patterns will significantly contribute to pave the way for individualised therapy [55, 116–118].

Most pharmaceutical companies now have recognised the need to implement biomarker discovery strategies as early as possible to advance the drug development process [119, 120]. It is expected that biomarkers can predict the outcome of late stage clinical trials with a high degree of certainty early in the process. In the future, biomarkers will play an important role in drug safety and efficacy measurements as well as for identification of inter-individual variations in drug responses [121]. The most important specimens for these purposes are readily accessible clinical sample sources such as blood, urine, or cerebrospinal fluid, which represent a major link between cells, tissues, and organs. When assessing these samples, in many cases, the crucial factor is not the detection technology, but rather the kind, quality, and quantity of the samples, with blood being the most difficult of all samples to analyse due to its intrinsic complexity [57].

Peptides proved as valuable biomarkers for numerous important indications already. Insulin and its by-products released during hormone processing are used to diagnose diabetes, BNP is applied for evaluation of chronic heart failure in children [122] and interestingly both, insulin and BNP are also used as therapeutic agents. Procalcitonin is the current gold standard for diagnosis of sepsis. In Alzheimer's disease, the beta-amyloid peptide is used to monitor therapeutic success by indicating the status of amyloid and plaque formation [116, 123]. Oncology is probably the most important indication for the application of peptidomics [6, 9, 124, 125]. Peptide expression profiling proved to be a highly useful approach to assess cancer heterogeneity and prognosis, and to indicate the therapeutic success of oncologic drugs. Furthermore, peptides derived from tumour cells are potentially useful markers in the early detection of cancer [126].

3.4.5 Indications

Our investigation revealed that R&D experts favoured the role of peptidomics in oncology, metabolic, cardiovascular, and neurodegenerative diseases with a strong emphasis on oncology in all areas of drug development. This is in agreement with the current impact of peptides/petidomics on medicine, since peptides proved to play an important part in diagnosis and therapy of these indications already. The very high potential of peptidomics predicted for oncology clearly reflects the key role of peptides in antigenic presentation, cell proliferation control, and the metastatic process making them ideal targets of investigation to elucidate this complex disease.

3.4.6 Collaborative efforts

Quite a number of potent global pharmaceutical companies appeared to be actively involved in development of innovative drugs. However, one of the most daunting challenges faced by the industry is how to isolate the subset of potentially useful targets that exist among the thousands that are currently available. Also technological challenges such as delivery problems associated with peptide drugs, their instability *in vivo* and short half-life remain critical challenges. Costly and inefficient large-scale manufacturing and purification processes are, moreover, hampering market growth. Optimising peptide delivery inside cells, tissue, organs or body will require increased R&D efforts. No company can do that alone. Instead, medical innovation of today is a concerted effort of academia, biotechnology, and pharmaceutical companies. Within this "orchestra", biotech companies have become an important new player in innovation during the last 15 years; they have the inherent advantage of creating diagnostic and therapeutic innovations very efficiently and frequently pass their research on to larger pharmaceutical corporations. For large firms cooperation with biotech companies often proves to be a very cost-effective and rapid entry into technologies and programmes that are not available in the pharmaceutical company. Such collaborative ventures will be essential to implementing new and effective peptide delivery technologies, developing synthetic peptides with increased stability and half-life, and realising peptidomimetic molecules that duplicate the structural and functional properties of biologically active peptides.

Accordingly our investigation revealed that pharmaceutical companies without exception seek collaboration with biotech companies. The difference between companies appears to be rather the extent and nature of collaboration than the decision as to whether or not to collaborate. The extent of planned cooperation seems to be largely dependent on the size and complexity of the pharmaceutical company's own facilities in innovative technologies. The one extreme is represented by Hoffmann-La Roche. Hanno Langen (Hoffmann-La Roche) reported that most of the research in proteomics/peptidomics will be performed in-house – a statement that certainly reflects Roche's extensive research activities in the field of proteomics expressed by the large proteomics initiative launched in 2000 with an investment of 100 million CHF for the following years. The other extreme is the comparatively small company Tibotec (Johnson & Johnson), focusing on innovative HIV/AIDS drugs, which intend to source out all peptidomics activities. Most companies, however, consider themselves somewhere in the middle of these extremes; the nature of tasks that these companies want to source out to biotech companies varies largely depending on individual requirements and prerequisites. Within the extremely complex and extensive process of innovative drug development the in-house activities of different pharmaceutical companies obviously emphasise different indications and/or areas of drug development. Also, expenditures for the following 5 years for peptidomics seem to vary among companies, ranging from less than 100,000 USD to about 500,000 USD in our study.

3.4.7 Future challenges

The rising need for new therapeutic approaches and advances in genomics and proteomics have boosted demand for small peptide and peptidomimetic drugs even as human genome sequencing has provided considerable impetus to peptide research. The current assessment among pharmaceutical R&D experts revealed that peptidomics, a powerful and highly sensitive approach to study peptides, is already significantly contributing to drug development and it has a high potential to further invade drug development soon. Experts currently consider its role primarily as complementary to other "-omics" technologies. An important role for peptidomics within the next 5 years was predicted by most respondents for diagnostics, for the development of lead compounds, for the prediction of therapeutic success, and for the prediction of adverse events. As indicated by the R&D experts, further advancement in this technology will depend on the development of appropriate validation strategies, and finally, on the transformation of analytical results into applicable assay formats, which can be used in a clinical setting.

Interestingly, although peptidomics obviously plays a crucial role in all areas of drug development already, the technology is barely perceived as yet outside R&D departments of pharmaceutical industry. This became quite obvious during the conduct of our study; while the terms proteomics and genomics were very well known in marketing departments of all companies, the term peptidomics was usually completely new to personnel outside the R&D departments. However, current R&D innovations will penetrate the market in foreseeable future. Therefore investigations such as this one may indicate future trends and innovations in order to create awareness in pharmaceutical marketing departments. The knowledge of innovative approaches and their role in the developmental process at an early stage is a sine qua non for strategic marketing planning.

Acknowledgements

We would like to thank all participants of this investigation for their most appreciated expert opinion: Dr. Alfred Hahn, Ludwigshafen, Germany (Abbott), Dr. Klaus Krauser, Abbott Park, USA (Abbott), Dr. Gerhard Paul, Ludwigshafen, Germany (Abbott), Dr. Gerd Bode, Hamburg, Germany (Altana), Dr. Sascha Dammeier, Konstanz, Germany (Altana), Dr. Andrew Young, San Diego, USA (Amylin), Dr. Philip Hedge, Cheshire, United Kingdom (AstraZeneca), Dr. Jutta Reinhard-Rupp, Frankfurt/Main, Germany (Aventis), Dr. Eckhard v. Keutz, Wuppertal-Elberfeld, Germany (Bayer), Dr. Martin Lenter, Biberach, Germany (Boehringer), Dr. Guido Grandi, Siena, Italy (Chiron Behring), Dr. Hiroyuki Kato, Ibaraki, Japan (Eisai), Dr. Bruce Pratt, Naarden, Netherlands (Genzyme), Dr. Peter Lord, Raritan, USA (Johnson & Johnson), Dr. Paul Guest, Harlow, United Kingdom (Merck & Co.), Dr. Vicente Nogues, Basel, Switzerland (Novartis), Dr. Frank Staedtler, Basel, Switzerland (Novartis), Dr. Klaus Rumpel, Sandwich, United Kingdom (Pfizer), Dr. Hanno Langen, Basel, Switzerland (Roche), Dr. Fujio Isono, Tokyo, Japan (Sankyo), Dr. Pascual Ferrara, Labege, France (Sanofi-Synthélabo), Dr. Nils Debus, Berlin, Germany (Schering), Dr. Serge Halazy, Geneva, Switzerland (Serono Pharma), Dr. Takanori Sato, Osaka, Japan (Takeda), Dr. Jaques Bollekens, Mecheln, Belgium (Tibotec).

3.5 Current Activities and Trends in Commercial Proteomics and Peptidomics Services

Ranald Sutherland

From a commercial viewpoint, the business of proteomics has evolved over a comparatively short time from a few players with a limited (service) offer, to many players with an extensive variety of commercial offerings and technology platforms. Some key trends observed are (i) the combination of multiple technology platforms to address the complexity of biology and disease phenotyping, (ii) a focus on smaller (bioactive) peptides, (iii) service offers to identify biomarker patterns/protein fingerprints and quantitation, and (iv) use of affinity binding technologies to enrich sub-proteomes for lead and target identification.

3.5.1 Targeting the need – pharmaceutical drug discovery and development

The pharmaceutical industry has the highest profitability of the Fortune 500, averaging profits of more than 18% of revenues, versus 7% for other industry sectors [127]. However, the high cost of R&D (estimated at ca 1 billion USD per marketed drug) [128, 129], long lead times to market (estimated at up to 10 years by the FDA), late stage attrition rates (less than 1 in 5 drugs pass clinical testing) [128, 130], and shorter patent protection periods (drugs with combined sales of 73 billion USD will lose patent protection by 2007) [131] puts pressure on pharmaceutical executives to find more efficient discovery platforms and development paradigms. Goldman Sachs estimated that the total R&D budget of the main pharmaceutical companies was 35 billion USD in 2001 [132], nearly double that of 1997 and triple for 1992. However the number of new medical entities (NMEs) submitted to the FDA has dropped each year from 34 in 1995 to 12 in 2003 [133], and the number of new drugs approved, from 53 in 1996 to 17 in 2002 [130]. A recent report from the FDA highlights the issues facing the pharmaceutical industry R&D process [130]. The report entitled *"Innovation or Stagnation"* focusses on the "increasingly challenging, inefficient and costly" medical product development process. A Tufts study calculates that improving the NME success rate in clinical trials from 1 in 5 to 1 in 3 could reduce R&D costs by 200 million USD for each drug successfully brought to market [134]. In an IBM study [135], 12 drugs with estimated peak sales of 11 billion USD were withdrawn from the market on safety grounds from 1997 through 2001. In addition, the pharmaceutical industry is being forced to re-assess the (so-called) "blockbuster" strategy where patients are treated in the same manner in spite of well-documented differences in response rates [135]. The drive to multiple and concomitantly smaller market segments is also the result of increasing use of genomic technologies to stratify patients, identify responders and avoid toxic side effects [136, 137].

In summary, there is a clear need to improve the pharmaceutical R&D pipeline efficiency and effectiveness. The FDA report highlights a number of areas with potential to improve the R&D process, including proteomics applied to safety assessment and adoption of new biomarkers or surrogate end points for effectiveness assessment [130]. This review paper focusses on commercial application of proteomics offered as a service. It should be noted that at present, the major proteomics market segments is in supplying tools/products to end-users. Examples include mass spectrometry systems, protein separation systems and protein chip technologies. Markets for proteomic approaches outside of pharmaceutical R&D are found in basic biological research, and industry research segments such as functional foods, where the main commercial players are Nestlé SA and Danone SA, and in the skin care market ("cosmeceuticals", e.g. L'Oréal SA). In these markets there is a need for biomarkers to support claims of product efficacy.

3.5.2 Proteomics services in the drug discovery and development value chain

The initial promise of proteomics was to support discovery and validation of novel targets, and to find new disease markers. A pioneer in the commercial service company were Oxford GlycoSciences PLC (OGS), which established a number of alliances in biomarker and target discovery with Pfizer, Inc. in Alzheimer's disease [138] and with Bayer AG for target discovery in respiratory diseases [139] (OGS were acquired by Celltech PLC in 2003 [140]). Today, there are many different proteomic commercial offerings. For the purposes of this review, these are basically classified by reference to the commercial need. This review also uses commercial case studies to highlight where the industry sees value, and also raises some key non-technical issues to be resolved in order to fully exploit the potential of the proteomics service business.

Target discovery and validation: In general the approach taken is to analyse tissue samples to identify which proteins are differentially expressed between diseased and control samples. Recently Abbott Laboratories, Inc. and Celera Genomics Group formed a strategic collaboration to discover, develop and commercialize therapeutic antibodies and small molecule drugs against over-expressed cell-surface proteins associated with cancer through proteomics research [141]. An alliance with similar goals was announced between (Biogen) IDEC, Inc. and Caprion Pharmaceuticals, Inc. for novel antigen targets for cancer therapeutics [142].

Protein interactions: The main commercial offerings focus on identifying protein-protein interactions based on the yeast 2-hybrid system (Y2H), a technology which has been in use for more than a decade [143]. Myriad Genetics, Inc. developed an industrial-scale, high-throughput application of the Y2H system (ProNet™). The commercial goal of applying ProNet™ is to identify genes representing opportunities for therapeutic development by defining disease pathways through protein interactions. Myriad and Bayer Corp. have a research collaboration focusing on the discovery of gene targets and the development of new therapeutics to treat dementia and depression. The research programme was partly based on ProNet™ technology and was subsequently expanded into biological pathways involved in the cause of obesity [144, 145]. Other offerings of commercial application of Y2H technology include Curagen Corp.'s PathCalling® platform (http://curatools.curagen.com/) and Hybrigenics SA's PIM Technology™ (protein interaction maps; http://www.hybrigenics.fr/).

Pathway mapping: The value propositions here are: (i) to identify whether a (novel) target is involved in a disease pathway and/or (ii) identify protein pathways associated with drug activity and efficacy. Cellzome AG developed their technology platform "Pathway Expansion" to identify disease association of novel targets. Cellzome established research collaborations, partly based on pathway extension, with Johnson & Johnson Pharmaceutical R&D to clarify the mechanism of action of compounds under development at Johnson & Johnson [146]. Curagen Corporation developed protein pathway mapping technologies to identify drug pathways with the aim of identifying alternative drug targets. Curagen established pharmacogenomics collaborations with Pfizer, Inc. to evaluate compounds under consideration at Pfizer, including protein pathway elucidation [147].

Biomarker discovery: Recently, commercial activity has been applied in pre-clinical studies, for example identifying markers which relate to toxicological effects. Surromed, Inc. have an alliance for biological marker discovery with Merck & Co., Inc. to analyse pre-clinical samples using its integrated platform for proteomic analysis [148]. Caprion Pharmaceuticals, Inc. have an agreement with Wyeth to carry out protein profiling in a pre-clinical model [149], and an alliance with AstraZeneca, PLC for biomarker discovery in a pre-clinical model for pain therapy [150].

Clinical proteomics: Clinical proteomics may be defined as the comprehensive, large-scale identification of protein patterns ("fingerprints") of disease, subsequently applied to assessment of disease susceptibility and prevention, individualised therapy, and monitoring of treatment response [151]. BioVisioN AG with their Peptidomics™ technology platform (www.biovision-discovery.de) and Surromed, Inc. with their Biomarker Discovery Laboratory (www.surromed.com) are positioned in this market.

Protein structures: An example of applying protein structural analysis to pharmaceutical research are Structural GenomiX, Inc. (SGX) with their technology platform FAST™ (Fragments of Active Structures) applied to lead compound discovery. SGX have an agreement with Serono Labs SA to apply FAST™ to generate novel lead compounds for selected kinase and phosphatase targets provided by Serono [152].

Database mining for novel proteins: An example here is the collaboration between Serono Labs SA and Inpharmatica Ltd. for the discovery of novel therapeutic proteins and drug targets. Inpharmatica applied their PharmaCarta™ technology platform to deliver sequences of more than 100 novel proteins to Serono [153]. PharmaCarta™ is an integrated suite of informatics based discovery technologies including Biopendium™, a proteome annotation resource which, in this case, was applied to data mining for small proteins.

3.5.3 Trends in pharmaceutical R&D that drive the proteomics service market

Some major trends in this service market include the following:

Disease markers: A significant change in focus is the move from targets to disease markers for many proteomic service companies. This is partly a result of improved technologies making a quantitative approach technically feasible. Other trends are, to focus on the shorter peptides, as this is where companies expect to find valuable proteins, and from single marker discovery to protein/peptide patterns or "clinical proteomics". Two commercial examples are BioVisioN AG's Peptidomics™ platform (www.biovision-discovery.de) and GeneProt's MicroProt™ platform (www.geneprot.com). As noted previously, there is considerable focus on toxicology markers particularly in the pre-clinical area. Another major trend is the move to bio-fluid analysis for biomarkers, including plasma and CSF. A key issue for commercial success with bio-fluids is to define reference methods and standardisation. This is reflected in the establishment of international co-operations like the Human Plasma Proteome Organisation (www.hupo.org).

Systems biology: The statistics of compound attrition rates indicate that the current drug discovery process is unable to identify lead candidates with a high probability of efficacy. The current "reductionist" approach such as used in high-throughput screening can not address the complex physiology and multiple causality of many diseases. There is a need for systems approach to biological research, which reflects actual working at the cell, organ or whole organism, and ultimately the pathophysiology of a particular disease state. Recent reviews emphasise a phenotypic approach at a biology system level to identify disease relevant targets [154, 155]. In attempting to address this need, there is a trend for companies to offer multiple, integrated technology platforms including proteomics, genomics, transcriptomics, and metabonomics linked together by a strong bioinformatics capability. Commercial proponents of this approach include Beyond Genomics, Inc. (www.bg-medicine.com) and Paradigm Genetics, Inc (www.icoria.com).

Personalised medicine: Personalised or targetted medicine has been described as the move from "one-size-fits-all" to biology based individualised therapies. Here, there is a role for proteomics in biomarker (pattern) discovery, probably in conjunction with genomics or other technologies. An example is the service offering of Surromed, Inc. (www.surromed.com), whose mission is "to enable the personalised treatment and precise diagnosis of disease".

Fee-for-service/CROs: In the past two years, more companies have been established on a pure "fee-for-service" basis with the capability to carry out a Clinical Research Organisation (CRO) -type service, testing thousands of samples in a few weeks. An example is the joint venture between Charles River Laboratories, Inc. and Proteome Systems, Ltd. to form Charles River Proteomic Services, Inc. [156]. It is expected that more fee-for-service companies shall focus on this market including extension of the current service capability in existing CRO companies.

Clinical proteomics: The FDA report states that there is a lack of novel technologies for clinical drug trials and there is insufficient applied scientific work ("translational research") for new tools in this area, which in turn results in the failure of the majority of investigational products [130]. PhRMA has calculated that total spending on US Clinical Development in 2002 was 9.3 billion USD and the attrition rate was 80% (www.phrma.org). To improve the chances of success, there is a significant opportunity for novel biomarker studies applied to clinical studies. However, the conventional view is that for use in the clinic, candidate biomarkers should correlate with the clinical outcome, have a biological link to the disease mechanism and also reflect the efficacy of the drug therapy [157]. This implies a "validation" process that is lengthy, resource intensive and probably requires phase II (+) clinical studies to demonstrate utility. Also, given a trend to evaluate "fingerprints" or peptide patterns as opposed to single markers, it is unclear how to define an acceptable "validation" strategy, a key issue for commercial success. One approach is to make clinical proteomics services available to pharmaceutical companies and reference laboratories as a service. An example is the commercial arrangement between Correlogic Systems, Inc., Quest Diagnostics, Inc. and LabCorp® where Correlogic's proteomics pattern recognition technology for ovarian cancer detection (OvaCheck™) is offered as a service [158]. In addition, clinical proteomic technologies could be offered as a service to carry out analysis of patient populations for "post hoc" patient population stratification. In a recent review on the use of biomarkers in the clinic, a crucial aspect identified was that novel biomarker studies be evaluated "off the crucial review path of a therapeutic drug dossier" to encourage wider use of biomarker studies [121]. One challenge will be to move from pre-clinical studies to "clinical proteomics" to demonstrate value in the clinical development process, [121, 151, 159, 160] and deal with the complexity of regulatory and other perspectives, a key for commercial success in the service business [161, 162].

Looking into the future, an area with opportunities for commercial services is the application of "pull down" or "enrichment" technologies using affinity ligands to select particular protein sub-populations. Applications include both removal of undesired protein species and concentration on proteins of interest such as receptors or enzyme families [163, 164]. Although this is currently mainly a market for tool/product companies, there are opportunities for commercial service offerings. An example is chemoproteomics, to enrich "sub-proteomes" with a goal of finding novel targets and leads. Serenex, Inc. recently established a technology evaluation alliance with Aventis Pharmaceutical, Inc. to evaluate Serenex' chemoproteomic technologies for lead identification [165].

4 Outlook

Peter Schulz-Knappe
and Hans-Dieter Zucht

One century of peptide research resulted in an enormous wealth of information for drug development and clinical diagnostics. The old relation of one biological function or disease to a single gene, which can be measured by a single marker or treated by a single drug, is no longer valid. With an estimate of 20,000 to 25,000 protein coding genes in the human genome, a multiplicity of three to ten times the number of proteins is expected owing to variations during transcription and translation. Further post-translational and proteolytic processing leads to the generation of myriads of peptides in a peptidome. Peptidomics certainly covers a highly dynamic field of research to explore this new molecular terra incognita.

Peptidomics complements the analysis of gene expression products by including the group of native peptides for profiling of states of disease and health. Peptidomics can close the gap between the analysis of metabolites, termed metabolomics, and the analysis of proteins, proteomics. It therefore forms an analysis platform that is capable to link static genotypes with dynamic phenotypes.

The manifold function of peptides in the organism, their role as products of degenerative processes and their accessibility in body fluids make peptides a promising target for analysis. Since peptides bear a great potential as diagnostic markers and may even be important drugs for therapy, peptidomics is used as a tool for discovery and validation of biomarkers, drug targets and lead candidates.

At present, the peptidomes of most relevant biological systems have not been explored in depth, therefore we expect a high number of relevant biomarkers to be detected in the future. Especially to reach the ultimate goal of individualized medicine, peptides will be of increasing significance. Thus, peptidomics will be used in many applications not only in academia but also in biotech and pharmaceutical industry.

Clinical peptidomics is expected to play a dominant role in future biomarker applications. It can be defined as the systematic, comprehensive, large-scale application of peptidomics technologies to samples from clinical trials. A major goal is the identification of peptides indicative of diseases and disease processes, and the application of this knowledge to improve drug development, patient care and public health through better assessment of disease susceptibility, prevention of disease, selection of therapy for the individual, and monitoring of treatment response. The outcomes of such analyses are biomarkers for early and differential disease diagnosis, prediction of response or adverse reactions to a therapeutic principle and disease progression under treatment.

Similar to the progress of genome research initiatives, multinational efforts as well as individual efforts are expected to have a major impact on the development of the field. From the multinational side, the Human Proteome Organisation (HUPO) is one promising example. One mission of HUPO is to assist the coordination of public proteome initiatives aimed at characterizing specific proteomes. Besides the brain and liver proteome project, the plasma proteome project, currently in the late stages of its pilot phase, will have a major impact on medical research, with the effort to identify proteins in serum and plasma and their range of variation depending on age, ethnicity and physiological state (32). In further stages, disease related and population based proteomics projects will be performed.

Clinical biomarker research has introduced specific requirements and challenges. Above all, clinical research is performed within a certain regulatory framework, which defines quality standards. Clinical research is usually accompanying approval proceedings, which defines the manner how to deal with the analytical results. The multivariate profiling of thousands of analytes, such as a pattern of peptides, proteins or transcripts, leads to results which can be interpreted in multiple ways possibly leading to a conflict of objectives.

Up to now, proteomics and peptidomics studies tend to analyse sample numbers well below one hundred. Whether this is appropriate or just a reflection of the premature state and the costs of the technology needs to be considered. In principle, it can be expected that the highly dynamic changes in peptide concentration and the high diversity of analytes makes the analysis of equally high sample numbers necessary. As a variation from the theme, less powered discovery studies may be performed, where a selection of validation candidates is selected with the drawback that many of the candidates will turn out to be false positive. It will need careful analysis whether the use of larger sample numbers for discovery of high quality candidates is preferred over the more meticulous validation of tens or even hundreds of candidates from smaller trials. Further challenges arise from the large amounts of analytical and clinical data associated with clinical trials. The definition and construction of clinical databases and the use of powerful statistical and data mining tools has to support the biological interpretation of the findings and hypothesis generation.

Each application has specific requirements for biomarkers regarding sensitivity, specificity, and validation procedures. Those requirements of the pharmaceutical and IVD industry as customers challenge the performance of the multitude of existing discovery technology platforms. The FDA already anticipated this development with its recommendations for industry on pharmacogenomic data submissions (www.fda.gov/cder/guidance/5900dft.pdf) which is not referring to data from proteomic and multiplexed data at the time being. This recommendation is in recognition of the fact that decision making during the drug development process is already partially based on such data. Nonbinding recommendations are outlined for data to be submitted on "known valid biomarkers", "probable valid biomarkers" and "exploratory or research pharmacogenomic data". Due to the burgeoning implementations of proteomics programmes in the pharmaceutical industry it is very likely that an equivalent recommendation for multiplexed proteomics data will be published in the forthcoming years. We expect a future dominant role for peptides in body fluids and tissues as markers of disease.

- Peptidomics complements proteomics for in-depth analysis of gene products.
- Peptidomics bridges the gap between the proteome and the metabonome.
- Peptides are ideal biomarkers, bioactive compounds and products of protein degeneration.
- Many peptide biomarkers are still to be discovered.
- Peptidomics is a valuable field to improve drug development.

5 References

[1] Schrader, M., Schulz-Knappe, P., Trends Biotechnol. 2001, 19, S55-S60

[2] Schulz-Knappe, P., Zucht, H. D., Heine, G., Jürgens, M., Hess, R., Schrader, M., Comb. Chem. High Throughput Screen. 2001, 4, 207-217

[3] Karas, M., Biochem. Soc. Trans. 1996, 24, 897-900

[4] Schrader, M., Jürgens, M., Hess, R., Schulz-Knappe, P., Raida, M., Forssmann, W. G., J. Chromatogr. A 1997, 776, 139-145

[5] Heine, G., Zucht, H. D., Schuhmann, M. U., Burger, K., Jurgens, M., Zumkeller, M., Schneekloth, C. G., Hampel, H., Schulz-Knappe, P., Selle, H., J. Chromatogr. B Analyt. Technol. Biomed. Life Sci. 2002, 782, 353-361

[6] Tammen, H., Kreipe, H., Hess, R., Kellmann, M., Lehmann, U., Pich, A., Lamping, N., Schulz-Knappe, P., Zucht, H. D., Lilischkis, R., Breast Cancer Res. Treat. 2003, 79, 83-93

[7] Lamerz, J., Selle, H., Scapozza, L., Crameri, R., Schulz-Knappe, P., Möhring, T., Kellmann, M., Khamenya, V., Zucht, H., Proteomics 2005, 5

[8] Pusch, W., Flocco, M. T., Leung, S. M., Thiele, H., Kostrzewa, M., Pharmacogenomics 2003, 4, 463-476

[9] Villanueva, J., Philip, J., Entenberg, D., Chaparro, C. A., Tanwar, M. K., Holland, E. C., Tempst, P., Anal. Chem. 2004, 76, 1560-1570

[10] Baggerly, K. A., Morris, J. S., Wang, J., Gold, D., Xiao, L. C., Coombes, K. R., Proteomics 2003, 3, 1667-1672

[11] Hilario, M., Kalousis, A., Muller, M., Pellegrini, C., Proteomics 2003, 3, 1716-1719

[12] Howard, B. A., Wang, M. Z., Campa, M. J., Corro, C., Fitzgerald, M. C., Patz, E. F., Jr., Proteomics 2003, 3, 1720-1724

[13] Markey, M. K., Tourassi, G. D., Floyd, C. E., Jr., Proteomics 2003, 3, 1678-1679

[14] Mian, S., Ball, G., Hornbuckle, J., Holding, F., Carmichael, J., Ellis, I., Ali, S., Li, G., McArdle, S., Creaser, C., Rees, R., Proteomics 2003, 3, 1725-1737

[15] Neville, P., Tan, P. Y., Mann, G., Wolfinger, R., Proteomics 2003, 3, 1710-1715

[16] Purohit, P. V., Rocke, D. M., Proteomics 2003, 3, 1699-1703

[17] Slotta, D. J., Heath, L. S., Ramakrishnan, N., Helm, R., Potts, M., Proteomics 2003, 3, 1687-1691

[18] Tatay, J. W., Feng, X., Sobczak, N., Jiang, H., Chen, C. F., Kirova, R., Struble, C., Wang, N. J., Tonellato, P. J., Proteomics 2003, 3, 1704-1709

[19] Wagner, M., Naik, D., Pothen, A., Proteomics 2003, 3, 1692-1698

[20] Zhu, H., Yu, C. Y., Zhang, H., Proteomics 2003, 3, 1673-1677

[21] Hansen, M. E., Smedsgaard, J., J. Am. Soc. Mass Spectrom. 2004, 15, 1173-1180

[22] Fayyad, U., Piatetsky-Shapiro, G., Symth, P., Uthurusamy, R., Advances in knowledge discovery and data mining, MIT Press, 1996

[23] Beebe, K. R., Pell, R. J., Seasholtz, M. B., Chemometrics: A Practical Guide, Wiley, New York, 1998

[24] Jackson, J. E., A User's Guide to Principal Components, Wiley, New York, 1991

[25] Malinowski, E. R., Factor Analysis in Chemistry, 2nd Edition, Wiley, New York, 1991

[26] Sachs, L., Angewandte Statistik, Springer Verlag, Berlin-Heidelberg, 1999

[27] Kitano, H., Science 2002, 295, 1662-1664

[28] Mohring, T., Kellmann, M., Jurgens, M., Schrader, M., J. Mass Spectrom. 2005, 40, 214-226

[29] Yates, J. R., III, J. Mass Spectrom. 1998, 33, 1-19

[30] Perkins, D. N., Pappin, D. J., Creasy, D. M., Cottrell, J. S., Electrophoresis 1999, 20, 3551-3567

[31] Bienvenut, W. V., Deon, C., Pasquarello, C., Campbell, J. M., Sanchez, J. C., Vestal, M. L., Hochstrasser, D. F., Proteomics 2002, 2, 868-876

[32] Medzihradszky, K. F., Campbell, J. M., Baldwin, M. A., Falick, A. M., Juhasz, P., Vestal, M. L., Burlingame, A. L., Anal. Chem. **2000**, 72, 552-558

[33] Chernushevich, I. V., Loboda, A. V., Thomson, B. A., J. Mass Spectrom. **2001**, 36, 849-886

[34] Morris, H. R., Paxton, T., Dell, A., Langhorne, J., Berg, M., Bordoli, R. S., Hoyes, J., Bateman, R. H., Rapid Commun. Mass Spectrom. **1996**, 10, 889-896

[35] Malmstrom, J., Larsen, K., Malmstrom, L., Tufvesson, E., Parker, K., Marchese, J., Williamson, B., Patterson, D., Martin, S., Juhasz, P., Westergren-Thorsson, G., Marko-Varga, G., Electrophoresis **2003**, 24, 3806-3814

[36] Lim, H., Eng, J., Yates, J. R., III, Tollaksen, S. L., Giometti, C. S., Holden, J. F., Adams, M. W., Reich, C. I., Olsen, G. J., Hays, L. G., J. Am. Soc. Mass Spectrom. **2003**, 14, 957-970

[37] Ross, P., Huang, Y. N., Marchese, J. N., Williamson, B., Parker, K., Hattan, S., Khainovski, N., Pillai, S., Dey, S., Daniels, S., Purkayastha, S., Juhasz, P., Martin, S., Bartlet-Jones, M., He, F., Jacobson, A., Pappin, D., J. Mol. Cell. Proteomics **2004**, 3, 1154-1169

[38] Keough, T., Youngquist, R. S., Lacey, M. P., Anal. Chem. **2003**, 75, 156A-165A

[39] Bogdanov, B., Smith, R. D., Mass Spectrom. Rev. **2005**, 24, 168-200

[40] Takada, K., Kanatsuka, A., Tokuyama, Y., Yagui, K., Nishimura, M., Saito, Y., Makino, H., Diabetes Res. Clin. Pract. **1996**, 33, 153-158

[41] Frederiks, J. A., Koehler, P. J., J. Hist. Neurosci. **1997**, 6, 147-153

[42] Pearce, J. M., J. Neurol. Neurosurg. Psychiatry **1994**, 57, 179

[43] Sakula, A. J. R., Coll. Physicians Lond. **1991**, 25, 171-175

[44] Toison, J., Lenoble, E., C. R. Soc. Biol. **1891**, 43, 373-379

[45] Pandy, K., Neurol. Centralblatt **1910**, 29, 915-919

[46] Lange, C. F. A., Über die Ausflockung von Goldsol durch Liquor cerebrospinalis. Berl. klein. Wochenschr. **1912**, 49, 897-901

[47] Kabat, E. A., Moore, D. H., Landow, H., An electrophoretic study of the protein components in cerebrospinal fluid and their relationship to the serum proteins. J. Clin. Invest. **1942**, 21, 571-577

[48] Schneider, G., Wallenius, G., Scand. J. Clin. Lab. Invest. **1951**, 3, 145-150

[49] Öhman, S., Quality assurance and sample handling in cerebrospinal fluid investigation. In: Cerebrospinal fluid analysis in multiple sclerosis. E. J. Thompson, M. Trojano, P. Livrea (eds.), Springer Verlag, Berlin, 1996, pp. 133-141

[50] Sanchez, J. C., Appel, R. D., Golaz, O., Pasquali, C., Ravier, F., Bairoch, A., Hochstrasser, D. F., Electrophoresis 1995, 16, 1131-1151

[51] Sickmann, A., Dormeyer, W., Wortelkamp, S., Woitalla, D., Kuhn, W., Meyer, H. E., J. Chromatogr. B Analyt. Technol. Biomed. Life Sci. 2002, 771, 167-196

[52] Yun, M., Wu, W., Hood, L., Harrington, M., Electrophoresis 1992, 13, 1002-1013

[53] Reiber, H., J. Neurol. 1980, 224, 89-99

[54] Reiber, H., Die diagnostische Bedeutung neuroimmunologischer Reaktionsmuster im Liquor cerebrospinalis. Lab. Med. 1995, 19, 444-462.

[55] Zolg, J. W., Langen, H., Molecular Cellular Proteomics 2004, 3, 345-354

[56] Diamandis, E. P., J. Natl. Cancer Inst. 2004, 96, 353-356

[57] Anderson, N. L., Anderson, N. G., Mol. Cell. Proteomics 2002, 1, 845-867

[58] Tammen, H., Mohring, T., Kellmann, M., Pich, A., Kreipe, H. H., Hess, R., Clin. Chem. 2004, 50, 545-551

[59] Hohenberger, Roche Diagnostics GmbH 2004. Compendium: Urinalysis with Test Stripes. http://www.diavant.com/diavant/servlet/MDBOutput?fileId=945. 2004

[60] Thongboonkerd, V., Klein, J. B., Jevans, A. W., McLeish, K. R., Contrib. Nephrol. 2004, 141, 292-307

[61] Pieper, R., Gatlin, C. L., McGrath, A. M., Makusky, A. J., Mondal, M., Seonarain, M., Field, E., Schatz, C. R., Estock, M. A., Ahmed, N., Anderson, N. G., Steiner, S., Proteomics 2004, 4, 1159-1174

[62] Spahr, C. S., Davis, M. T., McGinley, M. D., Robinson, J. H., Bures, E. J., Beierle, J., Mort, J., Courchesne, P. L., Chen, K., Wahl, R. C., Yu, W., Luethy, R., Patterson, S. D., Proteomics 2001, 1, 93-107

[63] Thongboonkerd, V., McLeish, K. R., Arthur, J. M., Klein, J. B., Kidney Int. 2002, 62, 1461-1469

[64] Winer, N., Sowers, J. R., J. Clin. Pharmacol. 2004, 44, 397-405

[65] Moller, D. E., Kaufman, K. D., Annu. Rev. Med. 2005, 56, 45-62

[66] Grundy, S. M., Brewer, H. B., Jr., Cleeman, J. I., Smith, S. C., Jr., Lenfant, C., for the Conference Participants, Circulation **2004**, 109, 433-438

[67] Catalano, P. M., Kirwan, J. P., Haugel-de Mouzon, S., King, J., J. Nutr. **2003**, 133, 1674S-1683S

[68] Kershaw, E. E., Flier, J. S., J. Clin. Endocrinol. Metab. **2004**, 89, 2548-2556

[69] Pfützner, A., Kunt, T., Hohberg, C., Mondok, A., Pahler, S., Konrad, T., Lubben, G., Forst, T., Diabetes Care **2004**, 27, 682-687

[70] Drucker, D. J., Diabetes Care **2003**, 26, 2929-2940

[71] Holst, J. J., Deacon, C. F., Curr. Opin. Pharmacol. **2004**, 4, 589-596

[72] Kadowaki, T., J. Clin. Invest. **2000**, 106, 459-465

[73] Robinson, S. W., Dinulescu, D. M., Cone, R. D., Annu. Rev. Genet. **2000**, 34, 687-745

[74] Herberg, L., Coleman, D. L., Metabolism **1977**, 26, 59-99

[75] Pelleymounter, M. A., Cullen, M. J., Baker, M. B., Hecht, R., Winters, D., Boone, T., Collins, F., Science **1995**, 269, 540-543

[76] Zhang, Y., Proenca, R., Maffei, M., Barone, M., Leopold, L., Friedman, J. M., Nature **1994**, 372, 425-432

[77] Halaas, J. L., Gajiwala, K. S., Maffei, M., Cohen, S. L., Chait, B. T., Rabinowitz, D., Lallone, R. L., Burley, S. K., Friedman, J. M., Science **1995**, 269, 543-546

[78] Hillebrand, J. J., de Wied, D., Adan, R. A., Peptides **2002**, 23, 2283-2306

[79] Coleman, D. L., Diabetologia **1978**, 14, 141-148

[80] Naggert, J. K., Fricker, L. D., Varlamov, O., Nishina, P. M., Rouille, Y., Steiner, D. F., Carroll, R. J., Paigen, B. J., Leiter, E. H., Nat. Genet. **1995**, 10, 135-142

[81] Friis-Hansen, L., Lacourse, K. A., Samuelson, L. C., Holst, J. J., J. Endocrinol. **2001**, 169, 595-602

[82] Fricker, L. D., Berman, Y. L., Leiter, E. H., Devi, L. A., J. Biol. Chem. **1996**, 271, 30619-30624

[83] Che, F. Y., Yan, L., Li, H., Mzhavia, N., Devi, L. A., Fricker, L. D., Proc. Natl. Acad. Sci. USA **2001**, 98, 9971-9976

[84] Bures, E. J., Courchesne, P. L., Douglass, J., Chen, K., Davis, M. T., Jones, M. D., McGinley, M. D., Robinson, J. H., Spahr, C. S., Sun, J., Wahl, R. C., Patterson, S. D., Proteomics 2001, 1, 79-92

[85] Rolin, B., Larsen, M. O., Gotfredsen, C. F., Deacon, C. F., Carr, R. D., Wilken, M., Knudsen, L. B., AJP Endocrinol. Metab. 2002, 283, E745-E752

[86] Kim, J. G., Baggio, L. L., Bridon, D. P., Castaigne, J. P., Robitaille, M. F., Jette, L., Benquet, C., Drucker, D., J. Diabetes 2003, 52, 751-759

[87] Thorkildsen, C., Neve, S., Larsen, B. D., Meier, E., Petersen, J. S., J. Pharmacol. Exp. Ther. 2003, 307, 490-496

[88] Young, A. A., Gedulin, B. R., Bhavsar, S., Bodkin, N., Jodka, C., Hansen, B., Denaro, M., Diabetes 1999, 48, 1026-1034

[89] Nagakura, T., Yasuda, N., Yamazaki, K., Ikuta, H., Tanaka, I., Metabolism 2003, 52, 81-86

[90] Balkan, B., Kwasnik, L., Miserendino, R., Holst, J. J., Li, X., Diabetologia 1999, 42, 1324-1331

[91] Ahren, B., Landin-Olsson, M., Jansson, P. A., Svensson, M., Holmes, D., Schweizer, A., J. Clin. Endocrinol. Metab. 2004, 89, 2078-2084

[92] de Meester, I., Lambeir, A. M., Proost, P., Scharpe, S., Adv. Exp. Med. Biol. 2003, 524, 3-17

[93] Marguet, D., Baggio, L., Kobayashi, T., Bernard, A. M., Pierres, M., Nielsen, P. F., Ribel, U., Watanabe, T., Drucker, D. J., Wagtmann, N., Proc. Natl. Acad. Sci. 2000, 97, 6874-6879

[94] Gronemeyer, H., Gustafsson, J. A., Laudet, V., Natl. Rev. Drug Discov. 2004, 3, 950-964

[95] Cai, W., Hu, L., Foulkes, J. G., Curr. Opin. Biotechnol. 1996, 7, 608-615

[96] Reginato, M. J., Bailey, S. T., Krakow, S. L., Minami, C., Ishii, S., Tanaka, H., Lazar, M. A., J. Biol. Chem. 1998, 273, 32679-32684

[97] Berger, J. P., Petro, A. E., MacNaul, K. L., Kelly, L. J., Zhang, B. B., Richards, K., Elbrecht, A., Johnson, B. A., Zhou, G., Doebber, T. W., Biswas, C., Parikh, M., Sharma, N., Tanen, M. R., Thompson, G. M., Ventre, J., Adams, A. D., Mosley, R., Surwit, R. S., Moller, D. E., Mol. Endocrinol. 2003, 17, 662-676

[98] Furuhashi, M., Ura, N., Higashiura, K., Murakami, H., Tanaka, M., Moniwa, N., Yoshida, D., Shimamoto, K., Hypertension 2003, 42, 76-81

[99] Rankin, J. C., Watanabe, T. X., Nakajima, K., Broadhead, C., Takei, Y., Zoolog. Sci. 2004, 21, 173-179

[100] Treerattrakool, S., Udomkit, A., Eurwilaichitr, L., Sonthayanon, B., Panyim, S., Mar. Biotechnol. (NY) **2003**, 5, 373-379

[101] Yamada, H., Igarashi, Y., Takasu, Y., Saito, H., Tsubouchi, K., Biomaterials **2004**, 25, 467-472

[102] International Human Genome Sequencing Consortium, Nature **2004**, 431, 931-945

[103] Rawlings, N. D., Tolle, D. P., Barrett, A., J. Nucl. Acids Res. **2004**, 32 Database issue D160-D164

[104] Davidson, H. W., Cell. Biochem. Biophys. **2004**, 40, 143-158

[105] Pfützner, A., Kann, P. H., Pfutzner, A. H., Kunt, T., Larbig, M., Weber, M. M., Forst, T., Clin. Lab. **2004**, 50, 567-573

[106] McClenaghan, N. H., Flatt, P. R., Diabetes Obesity Metab. **1999**, 1, 137-150

[107] Ferrannini, E., Galvan, A. Q., Gastaldelli, A., Camastra, S., Sironi, A. M., Toschi, E., Baldi, S., Frascerra, S., Monzani, F., Antonelli, A., Nannipieri, M., Mari, A., Seghieri, G., Natali, A., Eur. J. Clin. Invest. **1999**, 29, 842-852

[108] Lazarus, N. R., Penhos, J. C., Tanese, T., Michaels, L., Gutman, R., Recant, L., J. Clin. Invest. **1970**, 49, 487-496

[109] Yu, S. S., Kitbachi, A. E., J. Biol. Chem. **1973**, 248, 3753-3761

[110] Steiner, S., Anderson, N. L., Ann. NY Acad. Sci. **2000**, 919, 48-51

[111] Baggerman, G., Verleyen, P., Clynen, E., Huybrechts, J., De Loof, A., Schoofs, L., J. Chromatogr. B Analyt. Technol. Biomed. Life Sci. **2004**, 803, 3-16

[112] Anderson, N. L., Matheson, A. D., Steiner, S., Curr. Opin. Biotechnol. **2000**, 11, 408-412

[113] Kochendoerfer, G., IDrugs **2003**, 6, 1043-1045

[114] Owens, D. R., Nat. Rev. Drug Discov. **2002**, 1, 529-540

[115] Parmar, H., Therapeutic Peptides in Europe. Finding Opportunities, Frost & Sullivan, **2004**

[116] Aebersold, R., Mann, M., Mass Spectrometry-Based Proteomics, Nature 422, 13-3-**2003**

[117] Davidsson, P., Brinkmalm, A., Karlsson, G., Persson, R., Lindbjer, M., Puchades, M., Folkesson, S., Paulson, L., Dahl, A., Rymo, L., Silberring, J., Ekman, R., Blennow, K., Cell. Mol. Biol. (Noisy-le-grand) **2003**, 49, 681-688

[118] Ilyin, S. E., Belkowski, S. M., Plata-Salaman, C. R., Trends Biotechnol. 2004, 22, 411-416

[119] Richardson, P. L., Curr. Pharm. Design 2002, 8, 2559-2581

[120] Walgren, J. L., Thompson, D. C., Toxicol. Lett. 2004, 149, 377-385

[121] Frank, R., Hargreaves, R., Nat. Rev. Drug Discov. 2003, 2, 566-580

[122] Latini, R., Masson, S., De Angelis, N., Anand, I., J. Card. Fail. 2002, 8, 288-299

[123] Blennow, K., Hampel, H., Lancet Neurol. 2003, 2, 605-613

[124] Sasaki, K., Sato, K., Akiyama, Y., Yanagihara, K., Oka, M., Yamaguchi, K., Cancer Res. 2002, 62, 4894-4898

[125] Sato, K., Sasaki, K., Tsao, M. S., Yamaguchi, K., Cancer Lett. 2002, 176, 199-203

[126] Petricoin, E. F., Ardekani, A. M., Hitt, B. A., Levine, P. J., Fusaro, V. A., Steinberg, S. M., Mills, G. B., Simone, C., Fishman, D. A., Kohn, E. C., Liotta, L. A., Lancet 2002, 359, 572-577

[127] Proteomics R&D Competition Post Genome-Project Era, MRG Inc., 2003

[128] Backgrounder: How New Drugs Move Through the Development and Approval Process, Tufts Center for the Study of Drug Development, B., 2001

[129] Bain Drug Economics Model, Windhover's In Vivo: The Business & Medicine Report, 2003

[130] Innovation or Stagnation, US Department of Health and Human Services, FADA, 2004

[131] Global Generics Guide, Datamonitor Inc., 2002

[132] Global Research and Development Insight, Goldman Sachs, 2002

[133] Healthcare Institutional Investor Conference, L. Crawford, ACOF, 2004

[134] Outlook 2003, Tufts Center for the Study of Drug Development, B., 2003

[135] Pharma 2010: The threshold of innovation, IBM Business Consultancy Services, 2002

[136] Global Regulatory Trends in Pharmacogenetics and Pharmacogenomics. Life Science Navigator, Ernst & Young LLP, 2003

[137] Murray, D. M., Pharmacogenomics in Drug Development, 2004

[138] Oxford GlycoSciences PLC Announces Extension of Proteomics Agreement with Pfizer. Press Release, 2001

[139] Oxford GlycoSciences PLC Announces Acceptance of Validated Protein Targets. Press Release, 2002

[140] Celltech Announces Completion of OGS Integration Process. Press Release, 2003

[141] Abbott and Celera Genomics Announce Cancer Therapeutics Collaboration. Press Release, 2004

[142] Colon Cancer: Antibody Target Discovery, Therapeutic Development. Press Release, IDE Pharmaceuticals Corp. and Caprion Pharmaceutical, Inc., 2002

[143] Auerbach, D., Thaminy, S., Hottiger, M. O., Stagljar, I., Proteomics 2002, 2, 611-623

[144] Myriad Genetics, Inc. and Baer Corporation Expand Alliance to Develop Dementia and Depression Therapies with New ProNet™ Technology. Press Release, 1997

[145] Alliance Expanded into Obesity in Addition to Dementia Pathways. Press Release, Myriad Genetics, Inc., 2000

[146] Cellzome Announces Research Collaboration with Johnson & Johnson Pharmaceutical R&D. Press Release, 2003

[147] CuraGen Establishes Pharmacogenomics Collaboration with Pfizer Companies to Apply Predictive Toxicogenomics and Drug Pathway Mapping Technologies. Press Release, 2003

[148] SurroMed Announces Extension and Expansion of Biological Marker Discovery Agreement with Merck. Press Release, 2004

[149] Inflammation: Pharmaco-Proteomic Analysis & Biomarker Discovery. Press Release, Wyeth and Caprion Pharmaceuticals, 2003

[150] Pain: Pharmaco-Proteomic Analysis & Biomarker Discovery. Press Release, AstraZeneca International and Caprion Pharmaceuticals, Inc., 2003

[151] Granger, C. B., Van Eyk, J. E., Mockrin, S. C., Anderson, N. L., Circulation 2004, 109, 1697-1703

[152] SGX Forms Drug Discovery Collaboration with Serono Utilizing Proprietary SGX FAST™ Lead Generation. Press Release, 2004

[153] Inpharmatica Announces Expansion of its Collaboration with Serono. Press Release, 2002

[154] Fitzgerald, D., Gromo, G., Scientist 2004, 18, Art. 36

[155] Lindsay, M. A., Natl. Rev. Drug Discov. 2003, 2, 831-838

[156] Kerr, E., Gen. Eng. News 2003, 23

[157] Biomarker Definition Working Group (NIH), Clin. Pharm. Ther. 2001, 69, 89-95

[158] Correlogic signs Licensing Agreement with Quest Diagnostics and LabCorp®. Press Release, 2002

[159] Roberts, J. P., Scientist 2004, 18, Art. 38

[160] Cottingham, K., Anal. Chem. 2003, 75, 472A-476A

[161] Fleming, T. R., DeMets, D. L., Ann. Intern. Med. 1996, 125, 605-613

[162] Katz, R., NeuroRx. 2004, 1, 189-195

[163] Chapman, T., Nature Drug Discovery 2004, 430, 109-115

[164] Humphery-Smith, I., Proteomics 2004, 4, 2519-2521

[165] Serenex and Aventis Sign Agreement. Press Release, 2004

Abbreviations

2D	two-dimensional
3D	three-dimensional
3T3-L1	mouse adipocyte cell line
ABRF	Association of Biomolecular Research Facilities
ACE	angiotensin converting enzyme
ACTH	adrenocorticotropic hormone
AfA	African American
AFP	alpha-fetoprotein
AngII	angiotensin II
ANOVA	analysis of variance
aP2	adipocyte lipid-binding protein
AP-FXIII	activation peptide of coagulation factor XIII
aPTT	activated partial thromboplastin time
AsA	Asian American
ASP	acylation-stimulating protein
ATIII	antithrombin III
ATP III	third report of the National Cholesterol Education Program expert panel on Detection, Evaluation and Treatment of High Blood Cholesterol in Adults
BNP	brain natriuretic peptide
BPH	benign prostate hyperplasia
BVN P1	BioVisioN volunteer 1
CAN	correlation associated network
CCI	controlled cortical impact
CCK	cholecystokinin
CEA	carcinoembryonic antigen
CNS	central nervous system
CPE	carboxypeptidase E
CRO	clinical research organisation
CSF	cerebrospinal fluid
CV	coefficient of variation
Da	Dalton (unit)
db/db	diabetic/diabetic (mice)
Dec-RVKR-CMK	decanoyl-Arg-Val-Lys-Arg-chloromethylketone an inhibitor of prohormone processing
DNA	desoxyribonucleic acid
DPD	differential peptide display
DPPIV	dipeptidyl peptidase IV
ECM	extracellular matrix
ED	effective dose
EDRN	Earyl Detection Research Network
EDTA	ethylenediamine tetraacetic acid
ELISA	enzyme-linked immunosorbent assay
ESI	electrospray ionisation
ESRD	end-stage renal disease
fa/fa	rats having a mutation in the leptin receptor gene
FAST	Fragments of Active Structures (trade mark)
FFA	free fatty acids
FMRF	Phe-Met-Arg-Phe peptide
FT	Fourier transformation
FXR	farnesoid X receptor
GIP	glucose-dependent insulinotropic polypeptide
GLP-1	glucagon-like peptide-1
GLUT	glucose transporter
HCT 116	human colon carcinoma cell line
HDL	high-density lipoproteins
HIV	human immunodeficiency virus
HPLC	high performance liquid chromatography
HT	high throughput
HTS	high-throughput screening
HUPO	Human Proteome Organisation
IAPP	islet amyloid polypeptide
ICR	ion cyclotron resonance (spectroscopy)
Ig	immunoglobulin

IGF-I	insulin-like growth factor-I
IL-6	interleukin 6
INS-1	insulinoma cell line
IRS	insulin receptor substrate
IVD	in vitro diagnostics
kDa	kilo-Dalton
KDD	knwoledge discovery in data bases
KK-K^y	agouti yellow mice; obesity and type 2 diabetes mouse model
LBD	ligand-binding domain
LC	liquid chromatography
LMW	low molecular weight
LOD	limit of detection
LPL	lipoprotein lipase
LXR	liver X receptor
μRP	micro reversed phase
m/z	mass/charge ratio (spectrometry)
M	mol/L
MALDI	matrix-assisted laser desorption/ ionisation (spectroscopy)
MCC-555	a novel thiazolidinedione
MCP-1	monocyte chemoattractant protein-1
MEROPS	information resource for peptidases, http://merops.sanger.ac.uk
MHC	major histocompatibility complex
MIF	macrophage inhibitory factor
MMP	matrix metalloproteinase
MS	mass spectrometry
MS/MS	tandem mass spectroscopy
MSH	melanocytes-stimulating hormone
MW	molecular weight
NCI	National Cancer Institute
NME	new molecular entity
ob/ob	obese/obese (mice)
OGS	Oxford GlycoSciences (company name)
OGTT	oral glucose tolerance test
PACAP	pituitary adenylate cyclase-activating peptide
PAGE	polyacrylamide gel electrophoresis
PAI-1	plasminogen activator inhibitor-1
PC	prohormone convertase
PCA	principal component analysis
PCNSL	primary central nervous system lymphoma
PEPCK	phosphoenolpyruvate carboxykinase
PhRMA	Pharmaceutical Research and Manufacturers of America
PIM	protein interaction maps
pM	picomolar
POMC	pro-opiomelanocortin
PPAR	peroxisome proliferator-activated receptor
PPRE	peroxisome proliferator-activated receptor (PPAR) response element
PSA	prostate-specific antigen
PTM	post-translational modifications
qTOF	quadrupole time of flight
RP	reversed phase
RT	room temperature
SCID	severe combined immunodeficiency
SELDI	surface-enhanced laser desorption/ ionisation (spectrometry)
SGX	Structural GenomiX (company name)
SKI-1	subtilisin/kexin isoenzyme-1
SPSS	a data analysis software
T2DM	type 2 diabetes mellitus
TAT	thrombin-antithrombin III complex
TBI	traumatic brain injury
TF	tissue factor (coagulation)
TGF-β	transforming growth factor-beta
Tif-1β	transcription intermediary factor 1-beta
TNF-α	tumor necrosis factor-alpha
TOF	time of flight (spectroscopy)
TZD	thiazolidinedione
UCP	uncoupling protein
Y2H	yeast 2-hybrid (system)
ZDF	Zucker diabetic fa/fa rats

Index

Editors' CVs

Dorothee Gaenshirt

PhD, Ass. Prof., is a co-founder of the Health Care Competence Center, Basel (Switzerland).

As the head of one of the leading research groups in prenatal medicine world-wide, Dr. Gaenshirt is an internationally recognised authority, having written over 100 publications in this field. Her research group received substantial international funding from the industry and foundations, including Genzyme Corp. and the US National Institutes of Health (NIH). Her current academic title is Assistant Professor of Reproductive Genetics, University of Basel (Switzerland).

Dr. Gaenshirt was a co-founder and CEO of Cell Search Biotech, a spin-off company with significant international patents and a commitment to the development of innovative technologies for prenatal diagnosis. For 6 years Dr. Gaenshirt was advising international pharmaceutical and biotech companies in the area of drug development and approval of innovative therapeutics. She is the author of numerous articles dealing with the assessment of innovative drug development approaches. Dr. Gaenshirt is a member of the European Medical Writers Association, of the American Association for the Advancement of Science, and the New York Academy of Sciences; she is a referee for numerous scientific journals.

Fred Harms

MD, PhD, Ass. Prof., is a co-founder of the Health Care Competence Center.

After a successful international career at Lilly, medac-Schering, and Merck, Dr. Harms was Vice President and Member of the Board of OncoScore (Novartis-Venture). He has more than 15 years of experience in the pharmaceutical industry, serving in various international senior management positions including Research and Development, Business Development, Global Project Management, Marketing and Sales.

Dr. Harms is an internationally recognised authority in the field of Classical and Innovative Health Care Marketing, dedicated to future concepts for DtC (Direct to Consumer), DfC (Direct from Consumer), Service Marketing, Economical Marketing, Political Marketing with a special focus on Compliance Management and Patient Empowerment. Within the last 5 years he gave more than 100 lectures, published 3 books and over 80 articles in this field. As a physician and biochemist he is a member of several key leading organisations such as the New York Academy of Science, the American Association for the Advancement of Science, various European Cancer Societies, the High-Technology Entrepreneur Post-Graduate Program and the Society for Marketing Advances.

Sven Rohmann

MD, PhD, has been CEO of BioVisioN AG, Hannover (Germany), since June 2003.

Before heading BioVisioN, he was founding CEO of Ganymed Pharmaceuticals AG, Mainz (Germany).

Previously, Dr. Rohmann held several management positions during his ten years at Merck KGaA, Darmstadt (Germany), which include head of laboratories performing cardiovascular preclinical research, international product manager for cardiovascular products, international marketing manager, business area manager, global head of strategic marketing, and manager of the business area oncology, and senior in-house consultant.

Before joining Merck, he practiced as medical doctor at the 2nd Medical Clinic of the Johannes Gutenberg University, Mainz (Germany). Dr. Rohmann holds an MD from the same university and a PhD from Erasmus University, Rotterdam (The Netherlands), and has completed a post-doctorate research fellowship at the Max Planck Institute for Experimental Cardiology, Bad Nauheim (Germany).

His professional and managerial experience in the fields of medicine, especially cardiology and oncology, product management, strategic marketing, and business and corporate development in the pharmaceutical industry and research institutes gives him a strong base for developing new businesses in the life sciences.

In addition, since 2002 Dr. Rohmann has been a managing partner of Nextech Venture in Zurich (Switzerland).

He published scientific and business literature focusing on innovation management and marketing.

Peter Schulz-Knappe

MD, PhD, is a co-founder and CSO of BioVisioN AG, Hannover (Germany).

Prior to founding BioVisioN, he was head of department for preparative peptide chemistry at the Lower Saxony Institute of Peptide Research in Hannover. He was a member of the founding team of this research institute in 1989.

He studied chemistry at the Technical University of Karlsruhe (Germany) and human medicine at the University of Heidelberg (Germany) and University of Maryland (USA).

Dr. Schulz-Knappe started with peptide research during his MD thesis at the Institute for Anatomy and Cell Biology (University of Heidelberg) and completed his habilitation in cell biology at the Medical School of Hannover. In this work he conceptualised and realised the production of a human peptide bank from over 500,000 L of blood. This work led to numerous novel peptide identifications and formed the basis for the company concept of BioVisioN.

He published and co-authored over 100 papers for various scientific journals and is inventor of over 20 patents and patent families on peptides and analytical procedures.

The Authors

Annette Appel, PhD *
a.appel@biovision-discovery.de

Petra Budde, PhD *
p.budde@biovision-discovery.de

Prof. Dorothee Gaenshirt, PhD
Health Care Competence Center,
Birsigstr. 4,
4054 Basel (Switzerland)
and
EC Europa Campus
Bildung-Forschung-Innovation,
Balgerstr. 8,
76532 Baden-Baden (Germany)
d.gaenshirt@hc3.ch

Prof. Fred Harms, PhD,
Health Care Competence Center,
Birsigstr. 4,
4054 Basel (Switzerland)
and
EC Europa Campus
Bildung-Forschung-Innovation,
Balgerstr. 8,
76532 Baden-Baden (Germany)
f.harms@ch3.ch

Gabriele Heine, PhD *
g.heine@biovision-discovery.de

Rüdiger Hess, PhD *
r.hess@biovision-discovery.de

Marco Jost, PhD *
m.jost@biovision-discovery.de

Michael Jürgens, PhD *
m.juergens@biovision-discovery.de

Markus Kellmann, PhD *
m.kellmann@biovision-discovery.de

Jens Lamerz, PhD *
j.lamerz@biovision-discovery.de

Nicolas Le Yondre, PhD *
n.leyondre@biovision-discovery.de

Christoph Menzel, PhD *
c.menzel@biovision-discovery.de

Susanne Neitz, PhD *
s.neitz@biovision-discovery.de

Sven Rohmann, MD, PhD *
s.rohmann@biovision-discovery.de

Prof. Horst Rose, PhD
ImVisioN GmbH,
Feodor-Lynen-Str. 5,
30625 Hannover (Germany)
h.rose@imvision-therapeutics.com

Prof. Michael Schrader, PhD
Fachbereich Biotechnologie
und Bioinformatik,
Fachhochschule Weihenstephan,
85350 Freising (Germany)
michael.schrader@fh-weihenstephan.de

Martin U. Schuhmann, MD,
Assistant Professor,
Klinik und Poliklinik für Neurochirurgie,
Universitätsklinikum Leipzig,
Liebigstr. 20,
04103 Leipzig (Germany)
mus@uniklinik-leipzig.de

* BioVisioN AG, Feodor-Lynen-Str. 5,
30625 Hannover (Germany)

Peter Schulz-Knappe, MD, PhD *
p.schulz-knappe@biovision-discovery.de

Imke Schulte, PhD *
i.schulte@biovision-discovery.de

Hartmut Selle, PhD *
h.selle@biovision-discovery.de

Ranald Sutherland, PhD
Rue Daubin 22,
1203 Geneva (Switzerland)
evaranald@yahoo.fr

Harald Tammen, PhD *
h.tammen@biovision-discovery.de

Hans-Dieter Zucht, PhD *
*hd.zucht@biovision-discovery.de**

* BioVisioN AG, Feodor-Lynen-Str. 5,
30625 Hannover (Germany)